MENTAL
DISORDER

*An Introductory Textbook
for Nurses*

MENTAL DISORDER

*An Introductory Textbook
for Nurses*

H. Snell
R.M.N., R.C.N.T.

London
George Allen & Unwin Ltd
Ruskin House   Museum Street

Printed in Great Britain
in 11 point Baskerville type
by Cox & Wyman Ltd,
London, Fakenham and Reading

Preface

This book is written primarily for pupil nurses in hospitals for the mentally ill, and student psychiatric nurses in their first months of training. I hope it will also be of value to others whose work brings them into close contact with the mentally ill.

I have attempted to explain mental disorder in a way which I hope the reader will find meaningful and useful. To this end I have included a number of case illustrations, based on true life histories, but revised to be more concise and conceal the identities of the original actors. I have also included, wherever appropriate, suggestions for the general management and nursing care of the patient. The questions in the main text are designed to help the pupil nurse prepare for the final assessment, and provide the reader with topics for discussion.

The nurse will almost certainly be required at some time to care for patients who are mentally subnormal. The chapter on mental subnormality is included to give a broad outline of this psychiatric specialty, and to acquaint the reader with the problems of caring for the subnormal child.

Comments from students and teachers using this book will be welcome and should be addressed to the author, c/o George Allen & Unwin.

I am indebted to my friend Royce MacGillivray of the University of Waterloo, Ontario, for his assistance. I extend my thanks to Mr J. Churchill and his staff at George Allen & Unwin for their help in the preparation and publication of this book. Finally, I would like to thank Miss M. Wiggs who patiently typed numerous pages of the manuscript.

H. SNELL

Contents

	Preface	*page* 7
1	Past and Present Care of the Mentally Ill	11
2	Human Development	19
3	Mental Mechanisms and the Unconscious Mind	34
4	The Concept of Mental Illness	38
5	The Causes of Mental Illness	50
6	The Neuroses	56
7	Functional Psychoses	75
8	Organic Psychoses	98
9	Psychopathic Disorder	111
10	Drug Dependence	117
11	Epilepsy	133
12	Mental Subnormality	142
13	Fringe Problems	150
14	Aggressive and Suicidal Behaviour	159
15	Institutionalism	167
16	The Treatment of Mental Illness	174
17	Rehabilitation	190
	Index	198

Chapter 1

PAST AND PRESENT CARE
OF THE MENTALLY ILL

Mental illness has been recognised from the earliest times. Early Egyptian and Greek writings mention symptoms which today could only be regarded as evidence of mental illness. From the information available, we can assume that most illnesses, physical and mental, were at that time thought to have been caused by evil spirits.

From the darkness of those early years emerge the teachings of two great physicians. Hippocrates (c. 460–c. 377 B.C.) and Galen (A.D. c. 131–c. 201) refused to accept that diseases were caused by evil spirits. They taught that mental and physical disorders were caused by a disturbance in the body, and condemned the primitive 'treatments' usually prescribed for the sick. Instead of treating the mentally disturbed with confinement, flogging and starving, they recommended fresh air, relaxation and a suitable occupation.

Along with many other developments, the enlightened teachings of Hippocrates and Galen were forgotten during the Dark Ages. Almost nothing is known about the treatment of the mentally ill during those centuries, but we can assume that it reverted to punishment and the most primitive forms of medicine. Ignorance and fear continued into the Middle Ages, when mentally ill people were subjected to the most cruel forms of punishment and ridicule. The famous witch hunts of fifteenth-century Europe must have included many unfortunates who were mentally ill. Visions, strange ideas and odd behaviour were taken to be signs of possession by the Devil. Those who suffered in this way were hunted, tortured and often put to death by hanging, burning or drowning.

EARLY HOSPITAL CARE

The first hospital for the care of the insane in the British Isles began to accept patients in the fourteenth century. Known as Bethlehem, or Bedlam (a term used today to describe uproar) the hospital was originally a priory of the Order of the Star of Bethlehem, founded in London in 1247. For over 400 years it remained one of the few places of refuge for the mentally ill, but even there treatment was less than humane. Lunatics, who were not sent to Bethlehem and could not afford private refuge, were kept in prisons and workhouses. Some were cared for in hospitals for the physically ill, which were run by religious orders.

By the early eighteenth century, the mentally ill who had some money, or relatives prepared to pay for them, could be sent to private madhouses. The madhouses varied from small establishments able to accept 4 or 6 people, to large buildings which could house 200 or more. They were owned by private landlords who made a profit from accommodating lunatics. The madhouses were not usually supervised by doctors, and there were no nurses. The attendants were uneducated, and the patients were kept in appalling conditions, usually chained in dark, damp cells. The treatments were of the crudest kind, and included purging, enforced vomiting and blood-letting.

The madhouses were never inspected by any authority, and there were no restrictions on whom they could take in. They were often used by unscrupulous relatives to confine people who were not wanted, or so that their property could be seized. Many people were taken off to madhouses on some lame excuse, never to be seen again.

By the middle of the eighteenth century the conditions in private madhouses became a matter of public concern. Many appeals were made to Parliament, and in 1774 an Act was passed which ordered the licensing of madhouses and their regular inspection by Commissioners. This Act was an important step in a long chain of events which eventually led to the building of our present-day mental hospitals.

King George III (1760–1820) suffered several bouts of insanity during his reign. He was treated in a private house at Kew by a physician, Dr Wills. The treatment he prescribed was of little value and reinforced the opinion that something should be done to help insane people. In 1808 an Act of Parliament was passed which authorised every county in England and Wales to build its own asylum for lunatics. The cost of building, and later the cost of keeping the patients, was to be charged to local taxes. In addition, two justices had to sign an order before a patient could be admitted, and the asylums were to be inspected regularly. This Act provided, for the first time, at least some protection, care and medical treatment for the mentally ill. The first asylum to be built under the new Act was at Nottingham, and was opened in 1811. Other asylums opened soon after, and many were to become the earliest buildings on the sites of our modern mental hospitals.

DEVELOPMENT OF MODERN CARE AND TREATMENT

In the late eighteenth century, Philippe Pinel, a physician at the Bicêtre Hospital in France, embarked on a programme of improving conditions for his patients. Until this time many of them had been chained or kept in dungeons because they were so noisy and disturbed. Pinel unchained them, gave them work to do and freedom to move around. He soon found that their behaviour improved and that the whole hospital became a more peaceful place. His ideas were followed by many physicians in England during the nineteenth century. John Connolly, a physician at the Hanwell Asylum in Middlesex, and William Tuke of York, both dedicated their time and energy to improving the care and treatment of the mentally ill. Connolly was convinced that doctors and attendants should have a greater knowledge of mental illness, and devoted much of his time to giving lectures on the subject. In 1854 Dr Browne began classes to train nurses at the Crichton Royal Hospital in Scotland. Similar classes were soon to begin at other hospitals, and formal examinations for psychiatric nurses began in 1891.

Many laws were passed concerning the mentally ill during the nineteenth century, the most important of them being the

Lunacy Act of 1890. This Act compelled all local authorities to provide hospital accommodation for the mentally ill, and ordered that a person had to be certified insane before he could be admitted. The Act provided much better care for the mentally ill, but did not allow patients to be treated in hospital voluntarily. Although later laws improved the situation, it was to be many years before everyone could seek treatment without fear of being detained in hospital.

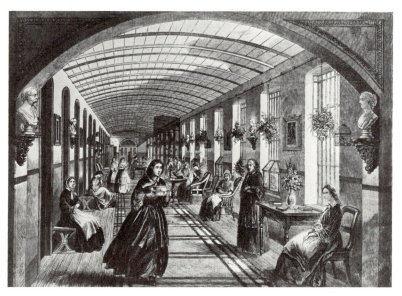

1 A ward in Bethlem hospital, 1860
Photograph by courtesy of the Board of Governors of the Bethlem Royal Hospital and the Maudsley Hospital

Despite changes in the law, and more humane care, mental illness was still surrounded by superstition in Victorian England. Mental hospitals provided refuge for the insane, but treatments remained crude and often ineffective. One most important breakthrough in the treatment of mental illness came at the turn of the century. It was discovered that the organism of syphilis could enter the brain causing the serious illness called General Paralysis of the Insane. It was soon found that high temperatures would destroy the organism and arrest the course of the mental illness. This was brought about by deliberately infecting the patient with malaria from a mosquito bite, and for the first time a major mental illness could be treated.

Following the success of **malarial therapy**, many psychiatrists became convinced that other mental illnesses had physical causes. In most cases, attempts to discover them have failed, but research has resulted in the introduction of some important treatments. In the early 1930s, it was found that by giving a dose of insulin large enough to produce unconsciousness, some patients improved. **Insulin coma therapy** was a widely used treatment for some types of mental illness until the late 1950s. Also in the 1930s it was discovered that by inducing fits artificially many patients recovered from serious mental conditions. The fits were first produced by drugs, but by 1938 electricity was used. **Electro-convulsive therapy** proved to be a highly successful treatment which is still used today.

Until the mid-1950s there were few drugs which could be used effectively in the treatment of mental illness. Bromide, chloral hydrate and barbiturates had been discovered earlier, and although they calmed the patient successfully, they also put him to sleep. In the early 1950s, the first tranquillizing drug became available. The drug was named 'Largactil', and it had the effect of calming the patient without making him sleep. Since then, a variety of tranquillizing and anti-depressant drugs have been manufactured, which have revolutionised the treatment of the mentally ill.

Along with the developments of physical treatments for mental illness, new and important discoveries were made in the field of human behaviour. Many of these discoveries were applied to the care and treatment of the mentally ill. Among the best known doctors in this field was Sigmund Freud (1856–1939). Freud devoted his life to understanding human behaviour and illness, and threw new light on the functioning of the mind in health and sickness. Some of his theories are mentioned later in this book, but basically he believed that all human behaviour and mental activity had a cause which could be discovered, if only people would search for it. As well as encouraging a greater understanding of the mentally ill, Freud has greatly affected the way we care for people in our society generally. In later years many famous doctors and psychologists have expanded on Freud's teachings, to give us an even greater understanding of our behaviour.

These important steps forward in the treatment and understanding of the mentally ill paved the way for greater freedom for patients in mental hospitals. In 1959 Parliament passed the *Mental Health Act (England and Wales)*, and in 1960 the *Mental Health (Scotland) Act*, which allow people to be admitted to a psychiatric hospital informally, just as they can be admitted to a general hospital. Many more people are now able to seek help for psychiatric illness without fear of being detained in a mental hospital. Today the majority of patients in psychiatric hospitals are receiving treatment of their own free will. The Mental Health Acts allow for seriously ill people to be detained in hospital against their wishes, but only under special circumstances and on medical advice.

Greater personal freedom for patients in psychiatric hospitals has developed during the last twenty years. With the exception of Special Hospitals, which treat patients who have committed serious criminal offences, most psychiatric hospitals now have few, if any, locked wards. Nurses no longer regard themselves as custodians, but members of a therapeutic team whose efforts are directed to meet the growing need for treatment of the mentally ill.

THE FUNCTIONS OF A MODERN PSYCHIATRIC HOSPITAL

In every psychiatric hospital there are, broadly, three groups of patients, usually referred to as short stay, psycho-geriatric and long stay patients. Short stay, or acutely ill patients are, with modern treatments, usually able to return home after a few weeks or months. Psycho-geriatric patients, or patients who suffer from mental illness in old age, form a large group in most hospitals. Many of these elderly people are able to return home after treatment, but some of them need to be cared for in hospital indefinitely. The largest group in most mental hospitals are the long stay patients. Many of these were admitted to hospital in the days before effective treatments, or have become so dependent on the hospital that they cannot easily leave. Many of them have a great deal of independence within the hospital, and help towards the efficient running of their wards and departments.

Patients are admitted to a psychiatric hospital, or a psychiatric unit attached to a general hospital, for different reasons. Some are seriously mentally ill, others have mild mental illnesses or are just unable to cope with the problems of life. Whatever their diagnosis, patients come to hospital because they need treatment, and can no longer lead satisfactory lives in society. The main function of a psychiatric hospital is to provide treatment which will help them return to a normal life outside hospital as soon as possible.

To provide the best treatment in the shortest possible time, the patient's life in hospital should closely resemble life in the community. The hospital must also be flexible enough to adjust to the needs of the individual patient, and to accept unusual or deviant behaviour without hostility, in a way which society is unable to do. This does not mean that the hospital should be without discipline. Rules are necessary here as everywhere else, but the patient must feel that he is free to express his feelings without fear of criticism. He must also feel that he has a share in the running of the hospital and in deciding his own future. Only if he is gradually encouraged to take his share of responsibility will the patient learn to adjust to the world which he has found so difficult.

A hospital which provides treatment for the mentally ill, allows freedom of choice and encourages patients to participate in their own treatment, is often referred to as a **therapeutic community**. In such a community the patients are treated, helped and encouraged by the therapeutic team. This team is composed of four main groups of people; psychiatrists, psychiatric nurses, psychologists and occupational therapists. Psychiatrists are doctors of medicine who have special qualifications in the diagnosis and treatment of mental disorder. A consultant psychiatrist is the doctor who accepts total responsibility for the care and treatment of his patients. Psychiatric nurses are trained to care for patients who are mentally ill. They work closely with the psychiatrists and other members of the team, and are involved in the treatment, care and rehabilitation of the mentally ill. Psychologists are trained to understand the reasons for people's behaviour. They are able to test patients to find out the reasons for their behaviour, and can supply the psychiatrist with important information. Very often psychologists are involved with special methods of treating the mentally ill. Occupational therapists play an important role in helping patients to relate to others through work and activity. They are able to teach new skills, and help patients to make better use of their leisure and work time.

In addition to these four groups of people, many others are involved directly or indirectly in the care of the patients. Social workers, pharmacists and hospital technicians provide important services, while hospital administrators, engineers and clerical workers help to organise and carry out the day-to-day running of the hospital. Only with a combination of individual efforts and skills can the psychiatric hospital fulfil its main function – the efficient care and treatment of the mentally ill.

QUESTIONS

1   Name three persons who helped to improve the care of the mentally ill in the past.

*2   Mention two main changes which have taken place in psychiatry during the last fifty years.

3   State one important change in the care of patients made by the Mental Health Act, 1959 (1960).

4   Name four groups of people who help to treat the mentally ill in hospital.

5   What do you understand by the term 'therapeutic community'?

* Reproduced by permission of The General Nursing Council for England and Wales.

Chapter 2

HUMAN DEVELOPMENT

Every human being is a result of the combination of two factors – **heredity** and **environment**. Hereditary factors are inborn. They are passed on from parents to child by tiny structures in the cells, called **genes**. Some aspects of a person, such as the colour of his hair, eyes and skin are entirely hereditary. Environmental factors are the person's experiences of the world, before and after birth. Education, personality, likes and dislikes are some aspects of a person which are almost entirely due to upbringing and experience.

Each person is born with a pattern for development, but this pattern is altered as he goes through life. Upbringing and early childhood experiences are most important, for they have a great effect on future development. Later experiences continue to change a person more slowly, but no less permanently, and these changes continue into old age.

As each person has a different heredity and grows up in a different environment, no two people develop exactly alike. Even identical twins, who have similar genes, develop different personalities in later life as a result of separate experiences. There are however certain stages in human development which are common to all. Every normal person who lives to old age passes through them, and each carries with it problems which must be dealt with. These stages of development are childhood, adolescence, adulthood and old age.

CHILDHOOD

Before birth, the baby is comfortably protected from the world. No demands are made on him; even oxygen and nourishment are provided without any effort on his part. Quite suddenly, at the moment of birth, he is thrust into a strange world, and for the first time experiences hunger, thirst and pain. Birth is probably the most painful and distressing experience in life. After it, the baby desperately needs security and nourishment, and demands them instantly.

A newly born baby sleeps a lot, and when awake is completely dependent on others for his needs. He cries when he is uncomfortable, but has no other way of asking for help. He soon begins to realise that, whenever he cries, someone cuddles or feeds him, and although he does not recognise that it is his mother, he begins to love the person who gives him so much comfort. Sometimes his mother may not be able to attend to him immediately, and for the first time he experiences the feeling of hate. All children develop a mixture of love and hate for their mother. This love-hate relationship is called **ambivalence**. As a child grows he must learn to wait for the things he needs, but for the young baby the learning is slow and difficult.

The child's mother expresses pleasure at the things he does by cuddling him, and her disapproval by scolding him. He soon learns to recognise the feelings in her and begins to need her approval just as much as his physical comfort. He will try to do everything to please her, and will be very upset if he does not get the expected response. Tears and screams follow when mother scolds him for bringing a 'present' of sand into her bedroom. To gain her approval he must learn to alter his behaviour, and remember the things she likes, and those she does not. This is an important and difficult stage of the young child's development. His mother should be constant in her reactions to him, and not confuse him by showing pleasure at his behaviour one day, and anger at the same behaviour the next. Confident, stable mothers generally produce well adjusted children. A child who is subjected to ever changing responses from his mother may grow up to be insecure, afraid and dependent.

MATURATION

When a baby is born, his brain and nervous system are not fully developed. This development will take some years to complete, and until then the child will not be able to do many things. Even simple skills cannot be mastered until he has reached a certain stage of development, no matter how much he is taught. This process of nervous development and changing behaviour is called maturation. The average child is mature enough to walk, and to learn to say a few words by the age of fifteen months. Even with careful training, bladder and bowel control may take two or three years to achieve.

FAMILY RELATIONSHIPS

The growing child's relationship with his mother is more important than his relationships with other members of the family. However, he has to come to terms with the fact that his father, brothers and sisters also have a claim to his mother's attention. He has to accept his role in the family and learn to get along with the other members of it. All this is very difficult for him at first. He will be jealous of his father's relationship with his mother, and will try to gain more of her love and attention by copying his father's actions. The child's relationships with his brothers and sisters will be particularly difficult. Sometimes he will be kind to them to please his mother, and at others he will be cruel and spiteful, because they are getting some of the attention he needs. The arrival of a new baby in the house can be very upsetting for a young child. He sees his mother lavishing her attention on the new member of the family, and feels rejected and jealous. He may react to this distressing situation by returning to an earlier stage of development. A return to bed-wetting, temper tantrums and 'baby-talk' is for him the only way of regaining some of the attention he has lost. This return to a more infantile way of behaving is called **regression**.

During the years when the child is learning to accept his role in the family, it is important that his mother does not show signs of rejecting him. He has to learn that he is not the only person in her life, although he will remain dependent on her for his physical and emotional needs. A child who is rejected at this stage of development may grow up to be anxious, insecure or aggressive. If a child is separated from his mother because she becomes ill, dies or leaves her family, the effect on him can be serious. He may become withdrawn, troublesome and less bright than the average child of his age. Not all children suffer in this way as a result of being separated from their mother, but in many cases the damage done can persist into adult life.

SCHOOL

Usually a child first goes to primary school at the age of five years. Unless he has been to nursery school, this is the first important break from his family. Most children take only a few weeks to settle down at school. At first, the emotion a child feels towards his mother is transferred to his school teacher. Junior school teachers are specially trained to help the child during this time, and realise the importance of his very early experience at school. A child who dislikes his first teacher may be unable to settle at school for a long time.

For the first few weeks at school the child is among strangers. He has a unique place in the family, but at school he is just one of a number. He must learn to find a new role at school and accept that other children are just as impotant to the teacher. This can be a great strain on the young child's powers of adjustment, particularly if he does not have a large family or is an only child. However, the more secure he is at home, and the more his mother has helped him to be independent, the happier he will be in his new role at school.

Play is a very necessary activity for children. It helps them to use up energy and learn more about the world around them. Until school age children prefer to play by themselves. In junior school classes children are encouraged to play together. Learning takes place gradually through play, but modern schools quite rightly place importance on the need for children to be able to relate to each other. Unhappy children who are not able to get on with others will not learn so quickly as those who feel comfortable in groups. Formal lessons and discipline are introduced slowly, and eventually the child becomes aware of the need to study for examinations. Parents can help the child to learn by providing opportunity to study at home and taking an active interest in his progress at school. Parents who expect too much from a child often find that his work falls below standard. This is because the anxiety they create in him, by expecting too much, impairs his concentration and performance.

The young child at school needs the approval of his teacher and companions just as he needs the approval of his mother. To gain this approval he tries to do well so that other children look up to him. Most children like to do well in sports and take pride in getting top marks in school work. Many belong to gangs at this time; another way of gaining acceptance and approval.

At the age of eleven years, a child leaves primary school for secondary education. In primary school he has been taught by one person for most of each school year. His companions are generally those children he first met when he was five years old. He may find secondary education very strange, particularly if he goes to a large comprehensive school. He will be placed in different classes for some subjects, and must get used to many different teachers. He will be expected to study hard for examinations, and will find that some teachers are more interested in his achievements than in him personally. Despite the sudden change of environment and personal relationships, most children quickly adjust to secondary school life without difficulty.

ADOLESCENCE

Adolescence is the period of development which occurs during the 'teens', and is a time of great physical and emotional change. For some young people it can be a difficult time, while others seem to pass through adolescence without experiencing many problems. Fortunately, most adolescents manage to deal successfully with their problems, and only a minority are seriously disturbed by them.

Puberty is the name given to the period of physical change at the beginning of adolescence. Young people grow quickly at this time, and both sexes develop **secondary sexual characteristics**. In boys, these are a deepening of the voice and the growth of facial and bodily hair, and in girls, the development of the breasts and the onset of menstruation. The physical changes are controlled by the secretions of the endocrine glands. These secretions also bring about sexual development, and have an effect on the whole body. Girls reach the age of puberty about twelve months earlier than boys, but in both sexes the time may vary widely. Some young people reach puberty at the age of eleven, and, for others, it may be delayed until the age of fifteen or sixteen. The most important changes in puberty are sexual growth and the development of sexual desire. The way in which young people react to them has a great effect on the emotional changes of adolescence.

The development of a healthy attitude to sex is very important for young people. All adolescents develop an attraction for members of the same sex, and this is a natural occurrence. Boys may be attracted to older boys, and sometimes form relationships with them. Very often the attraction is limited to the 'hero worship' of a famous football player or 'pop' star. Girls sometimes develop a crush on a female teacher or older girl. In most cases, this **homosexual stage** of development is followed by an attraction towards members of the opposite sex.

Emotional development can be hampered if the adolescent comes to believe that sex is dirty or unnatural. Young people usually relieve their sexual feelings by masturbation, and this can easily give rise to feelings of guilt. Many are led to believe, quite wrongly, that masturbation is wicked and can cause blindness or other dreadful diseases. Sex education in schools, if properly given, is perhaps the best way to clear up the misunderstandings which adolescents often have about sex. However, it is just as important to encourage healthy attitudes within the family. There is no doubt that many life-long sexual problems are caused by the unenlightened attitudes of parents and older members of the family.

The adolescent's relationships with his family can be very difficult. Teenagers are often hostile, argumentative and rebellious, particularly towards their parents. The reasons for this are easy to understand. On one hand, a young person is expected to be a man and become independent, and on the other, to be guided and controlled by his parents. He feels the need to be like older people, but is not emotionally mature enough to become independent. He needs his parents, but wants to break away from them. These opposing emotions make him feel angry, and the anger is usually directed at his parents. Later he will achieve his independence, and at the same time learn that he has a duty to his family.

In his striving for independence the young person needs the support of members of his own age group. He adopts the standards and interests of other teenagers, and involves himself in clubs, 'pop' music and dancing. Fortunately most adolescent activities are harmless enough, and only a few teenagers involve themselves with gangs, addictive drugs and crime. The overriding need of the adolescent is to conform to the standards and interests of his own age group. He can be accepted by others only if he wears fashionable clothes, uses the latest phrases, and adopts the life style and attitudes of his friends. Later in life the young person will be able to live more independently, form his own views and make his own choices. For the time being however his identity depends very much on the support he gets from other adolescents.

Many young people are very idealistic. They feel that they know what is wrong with the world, and how it can be put right. They naturally become angry and frustrated when their suggestions for a better society are dismissed or laughed at by people older than themselves. Many adolescents hold very definite views on issues such as politics, morality and religion. Very often their ideas and suggestions are desirable, but just as often they cannot possibly work. In late adolescence many people become disillusioned with the world. A few reject society and become 'dropouts', but the vast majority accept that the world changes slowly.

Except for those people who continue with full time education in colleges and universities, the first experience of working for a living occurs in the late teens. A few young people select a job that they like and are capable of doing, and immediately settle down for life. However, most people try several different jobs before finally deciding on a career. Personal relationships become more settled, confidence is gained, and the young person is prepared to take on a greater responsibility as he approaches the end of adolescence.

ADULTHOOD

Adulthood begins at the end of adolescence. A young adult is at the top of his physical and intellectual capacity. He is stronger than ever before, is able to work and become independent of his previous family. If he is emotionally mature he will be able to form more permanent, stable relationships with other people, and accept a greater degree of responsibility.

PERSONAL RELATIONSHIPS

If a person is to lead a reasonably happy and effective life, he must be able to relate to others. Furthermore, most adults feel a need to get along well with other people, to make friends and develop deep personal relationships. Some people are able to make friends more easily than others. On this basis people are sometimes divided into two large groups, the **extroverts** and the **introverts**.

An extrovert makes friends easily. He enjoys the company of other people, likes going to parties and dances, and engaging in sporting activities. He is a friendly, talkative person who prefers activity to sitting down and reading.

An introvert prefers to be alone, or with a few friends, rather than a large number of people. He would sooner read or study than go to a party. He is often thoughtful, hard-working and ambitious. Rather than choosing to have many companions, he will have a few, special friends whom he values highly.

Very few people are completely extrovert or introvert. Most are somewhere in-between the two extremes, having only a tendency towards one or the other. Whatever his personality type, a person needs to form meaningful relationships with others. To do so, he must be understanding and flexible in his approach, rather than demanding and intolerant. An emotionally mature adult will look first of all for what he can contribute to his relationships, rather than for what he can get out of them.

Most men and women eventually marry and have children of their own. Their choice of partner depends upon their earlier experiences in life. Emotionally immature adults are unlikely to form lasting, deep relationships. They may drift from one superficial relationship to another, always looking, but never finding, the security they desperately need. Some adults avoid deep relationships because they are always afraid of experiencing the difficulties and pain they felt when they were children. A few are still looking unconsciously for an ideal parent when they marry. This is often the case when a girl marries a man much older than herself, or when a young man marries an older woman.

Marriage is often held to be the ideal relationship between men and women. Young people may get married, thinking that at last they have found security, happiness and contentment which will last a lifetime. In most cases, this is far from the truth. Marriage, like any other situation, has its ups and downs, problems and disappointments. Work must be done, children must be looked after and difficulties must be met, long after the 'married bliss' has faded away. Young people who realise that marriage has its problems as well as its advantages are more likely to succeed in their efforts to achieve contentment. A stable marriage, or lasting relationship, is very important to the upbringing of children and the continuation of society. Even so, some men and women remain unmarried by choice, and are just as able to lead useful, satisfying lives.

RESPONSIBILITIES

All adults must accept a degree of responsibility, whether at work or at home with their family and friends. Most people have to work to earn a living. Depending on a person's choice of occupation and his education, work can be interesting and pleasurable, or monotonous and boring. There is no doubt that the job for which a man is best suited is one which interests him, rather than one which he does only to earn money. Whatever the job, he will be required to abide by rules. His attitude to work will be determined by his childhood experiences. If he was unable to come to terms with the authority of his parents and teachers, he will find it difficult to accept the discipline and frustrations of working life.

Some people find work difficult because they are unable to accept responsibility. They doubt their own ability to do a job properly, and the slightest criticism will make them give up. A child who was made to feel afraid and insecure may need constant reassurance and approval throughout his adult, working life.

There are some people who never seem to stop working. They go on and on, working long and difficult hours, taking more responsibility and seeking promotion. They buy larger houses, bigger cars and better furniture. They often excuse themselves by saying that they only work because they enjoy it. Certainly many people find enjoyment in work, but those who work non-stop, with little time for leisure, are driven by anxiety. They are worried that they will not do as well as the next man, like the child who needs to be at the top of the class to please his parents.

Despite the difficulties and frustrations of work, a suitable occupation can be a source of great satisfaction. Through work we are able to provide for ourselves and our families, and contribute to the society in which we live.

As a person goes through life, the experience and maturity which he gains help him to deal more effectively with problems. By middle age his own children will be growing up, or may already have left home. He will have many of the possessions he once sought after, such as a house, furniture and motor car. He is likely to be financially better off, and to have more time left over for leisure and enjoyment. For many people middle age is a time of security and contentment, without the worries of earlier years. For some people, particularly those who have always been anxious and insecure, middle age is a time of worry. They may look back on the past with the feeling that they could have done better. The future may not look bright, and they view it with fear and despondency. In women, menstruation usually ceases in middle age (the **menopause**), and they may become depressed with the knowledge that they can no longer bear children.

It is in middle age that people first give serious thought to retirement. Housewives never 'retire', and so the problem is really confined to men and unmarried women. Few people look forward to retirement with complete confidence. Even if they have no financial worries, they know that they will have to adjust to a completely different way of life after thirty or forty years at work. Sudden change is never easy, particularly in later life. Retirement can be made easier if the person plans ahead by taking up new interests and hobbies. Well adjusted people, who are interested in many aspects of life, seldom find difficulty when they arrive at the age of retirement.

OLD AGE

Old age has frequently been described as the time of life when a person declines physically and mentally. This rather gloomy picture is not always true, for many old people remain active and mentally alert until they die. The more severe disabilities of old age are caused by disease, and are not simply a result of growing old. There are, however, some changes which occur naturally in old age, and there is little that can be done to prevent them.

PHYSICAL CHANGES

Certain restrictions are inevitable in old age. Because muscles lose some of their power, elderly people are less strong and are unable to move as quickly as they once did. Their sight and hearing are less acute, and they may require spectacles or hearing aids. Blood circulation is slowed down, and old people have a dislike of the cold. Their appetite is reduced, and they prefer to take small, frequent meals. Many old people say that they are unable to taste and enjoy food as they once did. Because body fluid is reduced and the skin loses its elasticity, wrinkles and lines develop, giving an appearance of old age.

In addition to the natural changes, many physical diseases can occur for the first time in old age. Heart diseases, chest and urinary infections, rheumatic disease and diabetes are some of the more common illnesses of elderly people. Many of these can now be controlled by modern medical treatment. As a result, old people can expect to live longer, and remain healthier than ever before.

PSYCHOLOGICAL CHANGES

The psychological changes which occur in old age are less obvious than the physical changes. They may be mild or quite severe, but most old people develop them to some extent.

Old people like to **think and talk about the past**. They love to talk about the war and their experiences of years gone by, but find it difficult to talk about current affairs or the future. Very often they repeat the same stories, and seem to forget that people have heard them several times before. They **prefer the past to the present**. Many old people talk of 'the good old days' and are very critical of modern society, despite the fact that life today is generally more comfortable than ever before. They **prefer old ideas to new**. Many old people are suspicious of modern medical treatments, and some of them dislike modern gadgets such as vacuum cleaners and washing machines.

As people get old they **lose some of the ability to learn and deal with new problems**. This explains the difficulty many elderly people still have in using decimal currency, and why it is virtually impossible for an old person to learn to drive a car. In addition, they may find it **difficult to concentrate** as they once did, and this too makes it harder for them to learn.

Heredity plays a part in deciding how much a person will change mentally in old age. Some people alter a great deal, while others change very little, or not at all. People who have always been active and interested in the world around them stand a greater chance of remaining mentally alert well into old age.

PROBLEMS OF OLD AGE

For many people, retirement means a substantial decrease in their living standards. Unless they have made provision for retirement, or receive an adequate pension from their employers, old age can be a time of severe financial difficulty. Even those people who have managed to save a little money have seen the value of it dwindle with the inflation of the 1970s. Large numbers of old people find it extremely difficult to make ends meet. Frequently 'luxuries' such as holidays and entertainment must be given up in favour of basic necessities – food and warmth. Good food and heating are expensive, and some old people cannot afford enough of either. Sometimes these old people are admitted to hospital suffering from vitamin deficiency, or the effects of prolonged exposure to cold. In view of these financial hardships, it is a credit to elderly people that most of them manage to get by, often without complaining.

HELP FOR OLD PEOPLE

The government and local authorities are able to offer some help to old people in need. Some of the allowances and services they provide are:

Retirement pensions for people who have contributed to the government scheme while at work. Most working people have to contribute to the scheme by law, and therefore have a right to a pension when they retire. The pension alone is not large enough to live on.

Supplementary benefit for people whose income is not great enough to meet their needs. The amount of the benefit is worked out by assessing individual needs.

Pensions for people over eighty years are paid to those who have not contributed to the government pension scheme.

The pensions and benefits are given in a book of orders which state the amount of the allowance. The orders can be cashed each week at a post office. A person receiving a pension or benefit may have his allowance reduced if he spends eight weeks or longer in hospital.

In addition to cash allowances, local authorities provide **rate rebates** for people who are unable to pay the full amount of rates. **Free prescriptions** are available for men over the age of sixty-five and women over sixty. Certain other health services are also free of charge to elderly people.

Physical illnesses are very common in old age. The more chronic conditions, such as heart and rheumatic diseases, can mean that the person finds it difficult to get about, or is housebound. These illnesses can bring great hardship, particularly to those people who have previously been active. Relatives also can find the burden of caring for an elderly, sick person very difficult indeed. Nevertheless, it is important that old people be kept out of hospital if at all possible. Many old people do not like hospitals, and they will fare better if they can be cared for in the community.

If an elderly person is seriously ill or disabled, the government and local authorities can provide financial and practical help. An **attendance allowance** is available for people who need a lot of looking after by day or night. A **home help** may be provided to help with household tasks such as cleaning and washing up. The **meals on wheels** service can provide a hot midday meal at home if the person is unable to get one himself. Most local authorities provide a **laundry service** to help handicapped people with their regular washing, and a **home nursing service** for the chronic sick and disabled. **Health visitors** can make regular visits to the person's home to give help and advice on health matters. **Social workers** are able to give personal help to the elderly person and his family, and give advice about particular difficulties arising from illness or disability.

Many old people live alone and need a lot of support from the local authority services. Many local authorities run **day centres** where elderly people can take part in recreational and social activities. If an old person is unable to live alone, a place may be found for him in a **residential home**. These homes, which provide constant care and supervision, are run by local authorities and voluntary organisations. Many local authorities provide specially designed **council houses and flats** to meet the needs of elderly, disabled people. Some council houses for the elderly are supervised by a warden or nurse, who is available to give assistance to tenants if it is required.

Some old people lead very lonely lives. They may have no relatives or friends, or their relatives may live long distances away. The plight of lonely old people is sometimes mentioned in the newspapers, generally when an elderly person is discovered dead at home. Loneliness among elderly people is very common in the United Kingdom, for the needs and demands of the young are met more readily than those of the old. Only an increased awareness of our duties to the elderly will ensure that their needs are not forgotten in a fast changing society.

QUESTIONS

1   State two needs of a new-born baby.

2   Mention two ways in which a mother can affect the development of her child's behaviour.

3   What do you understand by the term 'maturation'?

*4   Give a common psychological reason for rivalry between brothers and sisters.

5   What do you understand by the term 'regression'?

6   Give two reasons why play is important for the development of a child.

7   What do you understand by the word 'puberty'?

8   Mention two reasons why an adolescent may disagree with his parents.

9   Mention one important psychological need of an adolescent.

10   State two psychological characteristics of a mature adult.

11   Give a psychological reason why a young person may marry someone much older.

12   State two advantages of middle age.

13   Mention three physical changes which occur in old age.

14   Mention three psychological changes which occur in old age.

15   Mention two problems of old age.

16   Mention two factors which affect the process of ageing.

17   State three ways in which the local authority can help old people in the community.

* Reproduced by permission of The General Nursing Council for England and Wales.

Chapter 3

MENTAL MECHANISMS AND THE UNCONSCIOUS MIND

In the previous chapter we have learned about some of the many problems every person must meet during his life. We may have concluded, and rightly so, that many human experiences are difficult, or extremely unpleasant. We may then ask ourselves what has happened to the feelings aroused by our experiences, particularly those of early childhood. Our memory of those early years is extremely vague. The feelings we had towards our parents, and even the way we were taught to control our behaviour, can no longer be called to mind. Have all these thoughts and feelings vanished without trace, or do they still exist, perhaps buried deeply within us?

Sigmund Freud, an Austrian physician, was one of the first people to suggest that early experiences do not disappear without trace, and he produced evidence to support his theory. He stated that the mind could be divided into three levels, the **conscious**, the **preconscious** (often called the **subconscious**) and the **unconscious**. The conscious mind contains all that we are aware of at any given moment. It includes our immediate thoughts, feelings and the awareness of our surroundings. The subconscious mind is comprised of memories, thoughts and feelings which we are able to bring into consciousness at will. When we try to remember what happened to us at some time in the past, we are really searching our subconscious mind for the information we require. The unconscious mind contains all the memories, wishes and feelings that we do not know about, and cannot recall even if we try. Much of the information stored in the unconscious mind is extremely frightening and unpleasant; for example, the hatred we felt towards our parents when we were very young. If these feelings and experiences were allowed to come into the conscious mind (in other words, if we became aware of them) our behaviour would become very disturbed and life would be impossible.

Freud suggested that a force exists in the mind which prevents us from becoming aware of unconscious information. This force, or barrier, between the conscious and the unconscious, he called a **censor**. Although because of the censor we cannot recall unconscious memories directly, they still exert a very powerful force on our behaviour. We do not fully understand the reasons for much of our behaviour, even though we like to think we do. In fact, almost everything we do is determined to some extent by the forces of the unconscious mind. For example, the girl who cannot settle in a job because she dislikes her bosses may **unconsciously** regard every boss as the father she disliked as a child. Unconscious memories sometimes come to light, although in a disguised way, when we dream. Dreams may be a way of releasing unconscious feelings which would disturb us if they were unable to find an outlet.

Although the unconscious mind governs much of our everyday behaviour, it seldom disrupts our lives. Fortunately most people are able to live with their unconscious. There is reason to suppose, however, that the abnormal behaviour of the mentally ill arises from the powerful forces of the unconscious mind.

As we have previously seen, mature adults generally respond to difficulties and stress by acting in a responsible and realistic way. Faced with an examination, most people will study hard in order to pass it. However, there are some problems which cannot be overcome by logical, realistic action. For example, being rejected by a friend or relative is something which cannot be easily dealt with. Faced with a difficult problem such as this, the normal human being uses unconscious psychological behaviour called **mental mechanisms**. Mental mechanisms are defences against anxiety, and help to protect the individual from anguish and feelings of helplessness. Because they are used unconsciously the person is unaware of them. Their use from time to time is a normal part of human behaviour, and helps to make life easier. If, however, this behaviour occurs more frequently than is necessary, the person may show symptoms of mental illness. Some of the more common mental mechanisms are:

Repression, or removing from awareness memories and feelings which are very painful. Like all mental mechanisms, repression is unconscious, and the person has no control over what is repressed and what is not. The disturbing experiences are pushed into the unconscious mind where they cannot be recalled at will. A child's hatred of his mother is one example of an emotion which is repressed.

Sublimation, or channelling unacceptable feelings into socially approved behaviour. Everyone has feelings and desires which are unacceptable, therefore sublimation is a widely used mental mechanism. The unmarried woman may channel her sexual energy into work for charity or dedication to her job. Aggressive people may channel their energy into playing football games or other competitive sports.

Reaction formation, when the person unconsciously deals with unacceptable desires by behaving in the opposite way to his true feelings. A married woman who is disturbed by her attraction to another man may state forcefully that she dislikes him. The person who strongly objects to hints of immorality in books and films may be disguising his wish to indulge in such practices himself.

Dissociation, which is an unconscious way of 'cutting off' painful experiences from the conscious mind. The man who is unhappily married may be unable to remember his married life. The use of this mental mechanism can produce symptoms of a particular mental illness (see Hysteria, p.60).

Conversion, or unconsciously changing painful feelings into symptoms of physical illness. For example, the girl who is afraid of marriage may become 'physically' ill in the weeks preceding her wedding. The engagement can then be broken off on the grounds of ill health. The mental illness which may arise from the use of this mental mechanism is discussed in Chapter 6, p.61.

Rationalisation, or unconsciously making up excuses for behaviour. The person gives acceptable reasons for the things he does and protects himself from the truth. The girl who always wears revealing dresses at a party may say that she can never find anything else to wear. The man who sits on numerous committees because he enjoys feeling important may state that he likes to help other people, or that he gives up his time because 'someone has to do it'.

Projection, or unconsciously shifting blame on to other people or circumstances. 'A poor workman always blames his tools.' The demanding, selfish girl will blame her boyfriend, and not herself, when he finally jilts her.

Regression, or a return to a more childish form of behaviour. When faced with a distressing situation, the person uses regression to relieve anxiety. Regression is generally seen in children, who sometimes return to an earlier stage of development on the arrival of a new baby in the house. However, everyone can behave in a childish way at times, and this behaviour usually annoys other people. The patient who is extremely anxious about hospital treatment may become completely dependent on the nurses, refusing to do even the smallest thing for himself.

QUESTIONS

1   What do you understand by the term 'unconscious mind'?
2   Give an example of how unconscious feelings affect human behaviour.
3   What is meant by the term 'mental mechanism'?
4   Name three mental mechanisms.
5   Give an example of regression in a psychiatric hospital patient.

Chapter 4

THE CONCEPT OF MENTAL ILLNESS

Ask a person who has no experience of the mentally ill how he expects patients in a psychiatric hospital to behave, and he will probably say 'They talk nonsense', or 'They do crazy things and can be very dangerous'. Even if he does not hold those beliefs about the mentally ill, he will almost certainly expect them to behave in a way that is very strange indeed. Certainly some patients do behave oddly, but the behaviour of most people who are mentally ill is not very strange. Many people who visit a mental hospital for the first time are quite surprised to find that the patients have a great deal of freedom, and that there are no bars or cells. Very often they will remark that, 'The patients look so normal'.

Whether a person is regarded as mentally well, or is said to be mentally ill, depends largely upon his behaviour. We often talk of 'normal' and 'abnormal' behaviour. Abnormal behaviour may differ from normal behaviour only in degree. For example, it is quite normal to become miserable at times, often with no valid reason. It is not normal to become severely depressed and think of suicide without good reason, and such a person would probably be mentally ill. Whether a person's behaviour is normal or abnormal also depends on his age, education, background and the standards of the society in which he lives. It would not be unusual for some South American tribesmen to dance around in a circle in the hope that it will rain, but such behaviour would be quite abnormal in a city office worker.

Some people do behave in an unusual way although they are not mentally ill. A man can choose to shut himself away from other people for months, in order to paint or write, and be perfectly sane. When a mentally ill person behaves in an unusual way, his behaviour is also likely to be out of character with his previous personality. For example, a quiet, thrifty, hard working man who never drinks is probably ill if he suddenly decides to spend all his money on buying drinks for other people in a bar.

Mental illness is sometimes described as a disorder of the mind. This description tells us very little, as the human mind is very difficult to understand. What is certain is that all mental illness causes at least some change in the patient's personality or behaviour. Psychiatrists and psychiatric nurses can only help a patient if they pay due regard to his behaviour, and what he says, thinks and feels. These aspects of personality are important clues to the diagnosis, care and treatment of the mentally ill.

THE SIGNS AND SYMPTOMS OF MENTAL ILLNESS

Mental illness can begin suddenly, or emerge slowly over a period of months or even years. If a patient suddenly becomes ill, it will be obvious to relatives and friends that something is wrong. If his condition develops slowly he may be very seriously ill before it is discovered. The signs and symptoms may be very mild, or quite severe and obvious to others. Few mentally ill people will have many of these signs and symptoms, and some may have only one or two.

GENERAL BEHAVIOUR

Sleep disturbance is very common in all mental illnesses. Some patients find it very difficult to get to sleep. Others wake during the early hours of the morning and are unable to get back to sleep. Difficulty in getting off to sleep, or in remaining asleep, is called **insomnia**. Sometimes mentally ill people sleep a great deal, or are only able to sleep during the day.

Loss of appetite (Anorexia) is another common symptom of mental illness. The person who normally enjoys his food may eat less, simply because he does not feel hungry. Other patients may eat very little because they are worried, miserable, too excited to eat or believe that the food is poisoned.

Personal appearance may be neglected. Some patients are unwilling to wash, shave, take a bath or change their clothes. A few dress in peculiar ways, or wear odd fashions or very bright colours. Very excited patients may not fasten their clothes properly, or refuse to wear many clothes at all.

Facial expression sometimes gives a clue to the person's feelings. A depressed person may look pale, drawn and miserable. Excited patients often have a ruddy complexion. Some patients look very anxious or lost, while others have odd facial movements and grimaces.

Interest in work, hobbies and surroundings may decline. A mentally ill person may give up work because he is no longer interested, or becomes unable to do the job. Some patients become so disinterested that they will lie in bed all day. Others may give up their usual interests for strange religions or peculiar projects.

Personal relationships may change. The person who was normally kind and considerate to his friends and relatives may become angry and hostile towards them. The friendly person may become withdrawn and refuse to speak to anyone. The person who was normally quiet may show an unusual interest in the affairs of others, or become excited and demanding.

ACTIVITY

Overactivity means a general increase in the patient's actions. The overactive patient does more, but he does not achieve more, because his attention wanders easily to other things. Mildly over-active patients are simply restless and unable to sit still. Patients who are seriously overactive move things around, hardly ever stop to sit down, and may become destructive. Often they cannot find time to eat or sleep because of their constant need to be doing something.

Underactivity means a slowing down of the level of activity. It is sometimes called **retardation**. The patient may find it very difficult to move around, to talk or eat. All his activities are painfully slow, or he may sit in a chair for hours without moving. Sometimes the underactivity is so severe that the patient lies in bed unable to talk or move. A state of complete inactivity is called a **stupor**.

Negativism means doing the opposite of what is asked. A nurse may ask a patient to remain seated in an armchair and he promptly stands up. Negativism does not mean that the patient is being deliberately unco-operative. It is a symptom of mental illness and quite beyond the patient's control.

Echopraxia is the opposite of negativism. The patient automatically copies the actions of another person. If the nurse stands up the patient stands up too. A patient who behaves in this way can sometimes become the centre of attention for other patients, and it is important for the nurse to ensure that he is protected as far as possible.

Echolalia means a repetition of whatever is said to the patient. The nurse will say, 'How are you this morning?' and the patient will reply, 'How are you this morning?', without answering the question. Echolalia sometimes has the effect of blocking all verbal communication with the patient, and it may be very difficult indeed to discover his true thoughts and feelings. Negativism, echopraxia and echolalia are most often seen in patients suffering from schizophrenia (see p. 79).

Compulsions are acts which the patient feels obliged to carry out, even though he knows them to be unnecessary or ridiculous. He may be compelled to wash his hands several times, or check that the doors are locked, even though he knows he has checked them before. If he does not carry out the acts he will become extremely worried that something bad will happen. Patients who suffer from compulsions always suffer from obsessions (see p. 44).

MOOD

A mood is a feeling, or emotional state, which lasts for a period of time. We are all subject to moods, and these range from great happiness and joy, to misery and deep sadness. The abnormal moods which sometimes occur in the mentally ill are:

Elation, or extreme happiness. Elation is an abnormal mood when it occurs without good cause. For example, the patient who is legally detained for treatment in a psychiatric hospital may be laughing, and stating that he has never felt better in his life.

Depression, which is really a state of extreme sadness. Depression is a symptom of mental illness when it occurs without cause or when it becomes abnormally severe or prolonged. The depressed patient usually looks sad, anxious and pale. He feels miserable, hopeless and is unable to enjoy any aspect of living. The future holds very little interest for him, and he is often preoccupied with morbid ideas. Communication with severely depressed patients can be extremely difficult, as they often find it hard to express their thoughts.

Inappropriate emotion, when the patient reacts with the wrong emotion to a particular event. For example, he may laugh when he is told by the doctor that he cannot leave hospital, or cry when a nurse tells him that a loved one is coming to visit him.

Emotional liability, or easily aroused emotions. The symptom is usually seen in elderly patients, or people who are mentally ill because of brain damage. A word from the nurse, a conversation overheard or a television programme may easily arouse laughter or tears. The nurse should be very careful not to say anything which may upset the patient, as even a chance remark may cause him great distress. Fortunately the emotions do not last for long periods of time.

Anxiety, or worry, which occurs to a certain extent in all mental illnesses. The patient is tense, worried or very afraid. He may find difficulty in sitting still, concentrating for more than a few minutes and in getting to sleep. Anxiety is a common experience in everyday life, but in the mentally ill it can become extremely severe.

Apathy, which is the patient's loss of interest in his surroundings and loss of his ability to show feeling. Apathetic patients show little or no emotional response to situations which would arouse normal people. They may sit for long periods of time, show no interest in work or leisure activities, and often neglect their personal hygiene. Apathy is a symptom of mental illness but it can also result from a lack of stimulation in the surroundings.

THINKING

Abnormal thinking is common in patients who suffer from the more severe mental disorders. It is often possible to tell if a patient's thinking is very disordered by listening to what he says and observing his behaviour.

Delusions. A delusion is a false belief which cannot be changed by logical argument. In other words, it is quite impossible to change the patient's way of thinking by arguing with him. Some deluded patients hold the most fantastic beliefs which could not possibly be true. Others have delusions which sound reasonable, and it is not unknown for them to convince others that their ideas are true. There are several types of delusion:

Paranoid delusions, when the patient wrongly believes that other people are plotting to murder him, trap him or annoy him in some way. Very often, the people who are after him belong to large organisations such as the Communist party, the B.B.C., the Roman Catholic Church or a foreign secret service. Quite often, paranoid patients invent a complex network of people and organisations who are plotting their downfall. Although their ideas may seem ridiculous to others, paranoid patients believe them to be true and often become very suspicious and afraid. Members of the hospital staff may become part of their delusions. For example, a patient may believe that the nurses are in league with his neighbours and the secret service, and are keeping him in hospital until he can eventually be murdered.

Delusions of grandeur, when the person wrongly believes that he is very important, wealthy or powerful. He may, for example, believe that he is God, Jesus Christ, a great historical figure or a member of the Royal Family. Patients who suffer from delusions of grandeur often behave in a very superior manner. They may refuse to talk to other patients or insist that they are being wrong-fully kept in hospital.

Hypochondriacal delusions, or delusions of bodily disease. The patient commonly believes that he has a disease such as cancer or syphilis, or that his bowels are blocked. Very often he is depressed, and believes that the imaginary disease will kill him before very long. Physical investigations and assurances from the doctor do nothing to alter his belief that he is physically ill.

Delusions of poverty, when the person wrongly believes that he has no money, property, or is in debt. Some patients will starve rather than accept food for which they believe they are unable to pay.

Delusions of guilt and unworthiness, when the patient is convinced that he has committed a grave sin and is not worthy to live. The patient will often say that he has sinned against God, and ought to be dead or burning in Hell. Patients who express delusions of this kind are usually very depressed, and often harbour ideas of suicide.

Nihilistic delusions, or delusions of death or non-existence. The person believes that he is dead, or that some part of his body is missing or has stopped working. Depressed patients may believe that they are already dead and being tortured in Hell. Patients who suffer from the more serious mental illnesses sometimes believe that they have no head, or that their insides are missing.

Thought blocking. This term describes the sudden interruption of a person's thoughts. A train of thought suddenly ends, and he may be quite unable to think of anything at all. Thought blocking can occur when a person is emotionally upset or very anxious. It is often seen in more serious mental illnesses when the patient stops talking in the middle of a sentence, or suddenly starts talking about a different subject.

Neologisms. A neologism is a new word. New words are often made up and used by patients with serious mental illnesses. Sometimes they use whole sentences of new words which sound like complete nonsense. When a patient who uses neologisms writes a letter he may include some new words which cannot be understood.

Obsessions. These are thoughts which come into the person's mind against his wish. He knows that the thoughts are ridiculous, but as much as he tries, he cannot get rid of them. Doubting that the doors are shut, or that the taps are turned off, or wondering why the moon stays up in the sky, are common examples of obsessions. Patients who have obsessions generally suffer from compulsions (see p. 41).

Phobias. A phobia is an unreasonable fear. Common phobias

are a fear of dogs, cats, spiders, heights and being shut in a room. The patient may be constantly worried that he will meet with the object or situation he fears.

PERCEPTION

Disorders of perception often occur in the more serious mental illnesses. The disorders are:

Hallucinations. A hallucination is a false perception which occurs without an external cause. Hallucinations can affect any of the five senses. The patient, who is seriously ill, may hear, see, feel, smell or taste things which do not exist in fact.

Auditory hallucinations, or hallucinations of hearing. These are the most common of the hallucinations. The patient hears voices which threaten him, use obscene language or give him instructions. Hallucinated patients may complain that they hear the voices inside their head, or they may be convinced that the voices come from outside. It is not uncommon to hear hallucinated patients shouting back at their voices, muttering at them or holding conversations with them.

Visual hallucinations, or hallucinations of sight. The patient has visions of people, animals or objects. Sometimes the visions can be very unpleasant or frightening. The patient may try to hide from his visions, stare at them with interest or become angry and abusive towards them.

Tactile hallucinations, or hallucinations of touch. The patient may feel insects or animals running over him, or strange sensations inside his body. Common complaints of patients with tactile hallucinations are of icy winds blowing over them, or of being sexually assaulted.

Olfactory hallucinations, or hallucinations of smell. Generally the smells are horrible, like gas or rotting bodies. The patient may complain of the dreadful smell, or insist that other people are trying to gas him.

Gustatory hallucinations, or hallucinations of taste. The patient has a horrible taste in his mouth, usually of poison. He may complain that people are poisoning him secretly, or give up eating because he believes that the food contains poison.

Illusions. An illusion is a perception which is misunderstood. The person sees something which is there, but in a distorted way. Illusions are very common in children, who often see objects in the dark as threatening figures about to attack them. A mentally ill person may, for example, see a cat as a tiger, or hear the sound of the wind as a machine about to destroy him.

MEMORY

The ability to remember events can be affected in many psychiatric illnesses. Patients who have been very anxious, excited or depressed are often unable to remember things that happened to them while they were acutely ill. Serious disorders of memory most often occur in old people who are mentally ill, and in patients who have received an injury of the head.

Amnesia means loss of memory. When a patient is unable to remember recent events, but can recall what happened years ago, the memory loss is called **anterograde amnesia**. Sometimes a patient may not be able to remember past events, but can remember what happened more recently. This type of memory loss is called **retrograde amnesia**.

CONSCIOUSNESS

Consciousness, or an awareness of the surroundings, becomes disturbed in some mental illnesses. Apart from unconsciousness, which is a complete loss of awareness, the following conditions are sometimes seen:

Confusion. A confused patient is bewildered by his surroundings. He may find it difficult to express himself properly, or be able to speak only a few words. Some patients become very upset and wander around, not really knowing where they are walking.

Disorientation. A disoriented patient, who is usually very confused, may not know the time or date, where he is or sometimes who he is.

CLASSIFICATION OF MENTAL DISORDER

Nurses may be surprised to find that their patients seldom fit exactly the textbook picture of mental illness. This problem hardly ever arises in a general hospital, where patients are physically ill. One case of appendicitis is very similar to another. The pain is about the same, in roughly the same area, and there are similar treatments for all. Mental illness affects the patient's personality. As every personality is different, mental illness does not produce the same symptoms in everyone. Neither will a treatment which relieves one patient necessarily be good for another. Nevertheless, certain types of mental disorder produce some characteristic symptoms. A classification along these lines will help the nurse to understand more easily the conditions from which many of her patients will suffer.

Mental disorder is the term used to describe all the conditions which may affect the mind. The Mental Health Act, 1959, defines four basic types of mental disorder. These are:

Subnormality, or inadequate development of the mind, particularly intelligence which requires special care or treatment.

Severe subnormality, or inadequate development of the mind, particularly intelligence, which is so severe that the person will always need care, and be in danger of exploitation by other people.

Psychopathic disorder, which is a disorder of character and personality. The person is irresponsible or aggressive, and it is considered that psychiatric treatment may help him.

Mental illness, which is described earlier in this chapter.

Patients who are subnormal or severely subnormal are generally cared for by doctors and nurses specially trained for this task. Those who suffer from psychopathic disorder are sometimes treated in hospitals for the mentally ill. People who suffer from mental illness, the subject with which this book is chiefly concerned, are treated by psychiatrists, psychiatric nurses and other therapists. Very often they are cared for in hospitals for the mentally ill and psychiatric units attached to a general hospital.

Mental illness can be divided into two large groups, the **Neuroses** (sometimes called **psychoneuroses**) and the

psychoses. The neuroses are generally milder forms of mental illness which laymen sometimes call 'nervous breakdowns'. The neuroses do not cause people to become 'insane' in the popular sense of the word. Neurotic patients realise that something is wrong with them (i.e. they have **insight** into their illness) although they may not know exactly what is wrong. The neuroses affect behaviour to some extent, but the behaviour of a neurotic person does not differ greatly from that of a normal person.

The psychoses are more severe forms of mental illness which affect the personality to a much greater extent. Very often psychotic patients do not realise that they are ill. Some of them live in a private world of their own and experience thoughts, emotions and sensations which we find difficult to appreciate. Their behaviour may become very unusual because of their strange experiences. The psychoses can be further divided into two main groups, the **functional psychoses** and the **organic psychoses**. Functional psychoses are those which have no known physical cause. Organic psychoses have a variety of physical causes (see The Causes of Mental Illness, Chapter 5).

A CLASSIFICATION OF MENTAL ILLNESS

   1 *The neuroses (psychoneuroses)*
- (i) Anxiety neurosis
- (ii) Phobic anxiety
- (iii) Obsessive-compulsive neurosis
- (iv) Hysteria
- (v) Reactive depression

2 *The psychoses*
A. Functional psychoses
- (i) Manic-depressive psychosis
- (ii) Involutional melancholia
- (iii) Schizophrenia and paranoid states

B. Organic psychoses
- (i) Senile dementia and pre-senile dementias
- (ii) Arteriosclerotic dementia
- (iii) Acute and chronic confusional states

QUESTIONS

*1 State some observations you might make on the mental
    state of a newly admitted patient.

2 What do you understand by the term 'overactivity'?

3 What is meant by the word 'delusion'?

4 Give an example of a hypochondriacal delusion.

*5 Give three reasons why a psychiatric patient might refuse
    food.

6 Give an example of an illusion.

* Reproduced by permission of The General Nursing Council for England and Wales.

Chapter 5

THE CAUSES OF
MENTAL ILLNESS

Unlike a bodily illness, which often has a single, proven cause, a mental illness can have a variety of causes. Some of the most common factors which may help to cause mental illness are mentioned here, but it must be remembered that many of these cannot be definitely proved.

A patient's relatives will often blame one factor or set of circumstances for his mental breakdown. Divorce, broken love affairs, bereavements and examinations are commonly blamed for mental illness. Finding a cause for the person's breakdown is not unnatural, for we all like to blame someone or something for our misfortunes. Unfortunately the causes are seldom so simple as this. Certainly broken love affairs and bereavements can help to cause mental illness, but almost everyone experiences one or the other at some time. Most people manage to get over these difficulties, and only a few become mentally ill as a result.

Except in a few cases, no single cause is responsible for mental illness. For example, a young man whose parents were always at loggerheads when he was a child became mentally ill just before his examinations at university. It would be easy to blame overwork and the stress of the examinations for his illness, were it not for the fact that his colleagues did not become ill. It is more likely that his upbringing, which left him insecure, made it more likely that he would become ill under stress. In this case two factors are responsible; his childhood experiences and the stress of his examinations.

In most cases the causes of mental illness are very involved and cannot be definitely proved. Nevertheless, it helps our understanding of the patient if we are able to discover some of the circumstances which have led to his breakdown. The causes of mental illness can be divided into three main groups. These are the effects of **physical disease**, **heredity** and **personal experience**.

PHYSICAL DISEASE

Any physical illness can produce mental, as well as physical symptoms. For example, influenza, as well as producing malaise, joint pains, headache, coughs and sneezes can, in some people, produce severe depression. However, the physical diseases most likely to cause a mental illness are those which have an effect upon the brain itself. These include:

1 Disease of the brain, e.g. brain tumour, syphilis, meningitis, reduction of blood supply to the brain and death of brain cells in old age.
2 Injury to the brain as a result of accident or a major operation.
3 Poisoning with alcohol, barbiturates, amphetamines and gases, or the toxic effects of severe bodily infections.
4 Bodily diseases which interfere with the functioning of the brain, e.g. heart failure, renal or liver disease, diabetes and vitamin deficiency.

HEREDITY

It is quite often said that mental illness runs in families. This may sometimes be true, but in the majority of cases it cannot actually be proved. Many patients have relatives who have been treated for mental illness, but generally this does not prove that the disorder is hereditary. Some psychiatrists believe that many of the serious mental illnesses are inherited, while others argue that the child's upbringing is the most important factor. Whatever the truth of the matter, only a very small number of mental illnesses can definitely be proved to be hereditary.

PERSONAL EXPERIENCES

Personal experiences are extremely important to the development of personality and to the way we learn to deal with our problems.

Their effect on mental health is best understood if we divide them into two groups, childhood experiences and adult experiences. As we have seen in the example of the young man who became ill just before his examinations, childhood experiences have a great effect on the way we deal with problems later in life. This is true, no matter what a patient's immediate difficulty may be.

CHILDHOOD EXPERIENCES

We have previously referred to some of the adjustments which a young person must make if he is to grow into a responsible, secure adult. Even the youngest child must learn to deal with situations which, at that time, are extremely difficult and upsetting. He must learn to please his mother, even if it means giving up something he likes doing. He has to accept that other people need some of his mother's attention, and he must learn to share her with them. These are difficult and painful times for the child, and he is made anxious and angry by them. The painful memories and emotions are eventually pushed from his mind by the process of repression (see p. 36). If something goes wrong with this process, the memories and feelings may continue to trouble him, and may result in mental illness later in life. His mother must also understand his feelings. If she always becomes angry with him, or threatens to reject him, she may easily inflict lasting emotional damage on her child. He may grow up to feel that he cannot trust anyone, and personal relationships will become a great cause for anxiety in him.

All parents have a duty to teach their children to tell the difference between right and wrong. This is the only way a child will grow up to be a responsible, respectable citizen. However, some parents have very rigid and old fashioned attitudes, and expect too much from their children. They demand a high standard of behaviour, and make them feel wretched and guilty if they misbehave. This guilt can persist into adult life, particularly if the person is unable to keep up to the standards set by his parents. Guilt is a very important factor in the cause of many mental illnesses.

When a child falls over and hurts himself, or becomes ill, he will turn to his mother for comfort and security. Most mothers give their children extra love and attention when they are sick. This is necessary because a young child is incapable of caring for himself. However, if a mother encourages her child to turn to her for comfort for the slightest mishap, she can do more harm than good. The child may learn that illness is a way of getting extra attention, and this behaviour can persist into adult life. Some people who are mentally ill seek love and attention through physical illness, and never become fully mature.

Children learn a great deal by example. They copy the behaviour of other children, adults, and more especially their own parents. In this way they learn good patterns of behaviour, and sometimes faulty ones. Parents who deal calmly and responsibly with difficulties are likely to teach their children similar patterns of behaviour. Those who become very anxious and upset by minor problems are likely to produce children who will eventually behave in a similar way. Anxiety can be learned in this way, and so can some mental illnesses.

Some mothers never let their children grow up. They protect them from every difficulty long after they should be able to deal with problems on their own. It is as if these mothers are afraid that their children will grow away from them. Very often a child who is overprotected will grow up unable to accept responsibility. Faced with difficulty he will want to return to his mother, and will often develop symptoms of anxiety.

All children have to deal with a multitude of problems. Fortunately most of them manage to do so successfully. Those who for some reason do not often find greater difficulty in dealing with the problems of adult life. A few of these may find life's problems so difficult that they break down with mental illness.

ADULT EXPERIENCES

Every person has to meet a host of problems during his adult life. Some of the difficulties which may be associated with mental illness are:

The problems of adolescence. The adolescent stage of

development (see p. 23), when young people must adapt to physical and emotional changes, often gives rise to stress. Mental illness often develops for the first time during adolescence.

Marriage difficulties. Marriage involves giving up a great deal of independence, leaving home and adjusting to a new way of life. Extra responsibilities must be taken on, and for some people the adjustment is very difficult. Mental illness sometimes appears during the first few years of married life.

Childbirth. Pregnancy, and later the problems of caring for a young baby place a great responsibility on a mother. She will have to give up work, at least for a time, to care for the young child. She may find that she has little time left over for leisure and entertainment, and she may quite easily become anxious or depressed. Sometimes the physical changes of pregnancy can help to cause mental illness, even in a mother who would otherwise be quite able to cope.

Stress at work. Many people like to blame overwork as the cause of mental illness. Certainly the stress of work can help to cause illness, particularly if the person is under pressure or takes on a high degree of responsibility. However, overwork is more often a way of dealing with anxiety, and is a symptom of mental illness rather than a cause of it (see p. 28).

The problems of middle age. Some people find the problems of middle age (see 28) very difficult to overcome. They feel that life is beginning to pass them by, and they worry a great deal about the future. Women, who usually cannot bear children after this time, may feel useless and dejected. Certain mental illnesses may occur for the first time at this period of life.

The problems of retirement. For many people retirement means giving up a life of interest and hard work, with very little to take its place (see p. 28). Men particularly may feel useless and unwanted at this time. Mental illness sometimes develops shortly after retirement.

Financial difficulties. People who become unemployed or suffer a financial setback often find that they are in debt. Financial difficulties can be very worrying, and some people break down with anxiety or depression as a result. This often happens when a person feels that he is to blame for his situation, for example when he has not been able to manage his affairs properly. Unemployment presents particular problems for a married man. In addition to his financial worries, he may feel guilty because he is unable to support his wife and children. Depressive illness can arise as a result of unemployment, particularly in people of middle age.

Bereavement. Mental illness sometimes follows the death of a loved one. This usually happens when the relationship has been very deep, and a great deal of love and security has been lost. The usual period of grief and mourning after the death of a loved one is not regarded as a mental illness.

Except in a small number of cases, psychiatrists and psychologists are only able to suggest the causes of mental illness. Whether through the effects of heredity or upbringing, some people react to the problems of life by becoming mentally ill. No one can be blamed for mental illness, least of all the patient himself. One fact is absolutely certain; we can all become mentally ill if we are subjected to stress which is severe enough. It can happen to us all, no matter how well adjusted and mature we may be.

QUESTIONS

1 Give two physical causes of mental illness.
2 Mention two factors in the upbringing of a child which may lead to mental illness later in life.
3 Mention one factor associated with childbirth which may help to cause mental illness.
4 Mention one factor associated with middle age which may help to cause mental illness.
*5 List two factors in an individual's personality or his environment which may contribute to mental illness.

* Reproduced by permission of The General Nursing Council for England and Wales.

Chapter 6

THE NEUROSES

The neuroses are a large group of mental disorders which are not severe enough to be labelled as forms of 'insanity' but yet are troublesome enough to prompt many sufferers to seek medical advice. The term 'nervous breakdown', much used by laymen, generally refers to this group of mental illnesses.

A number of people are said to have **neurotic traits**. This does not mean that they are mentally ill, or that they are going to develop mental illness. Indeed, it is quite usual for some neurotic traits to appear when a person is under severe stress. However, some people have a greater tendency to neurotic behaviour than others. The greater the tendency, the more likely it is that the person will produce symptoms of mental illness when life becomes difficult.

People with a marked tendency to neurotic behaviour are sometimes said to have a neurotic personality. Such a personality is difficult to define. Neurotic people tend to complain of more 'physical' ailments than normal people. Vague aches and pains, headaches, dizziness, palpitations, blurred vision, and stomach upsets are all common complaints of the neurotic person. Such symptoms have no physical cause, yet they are real enough to the patient.

Neurotic people are inclined to be more sensitive, more emotional and less reliable than normal individuals. They rely greatly upon other people, are often possessive and seldom independent. Frequently they are insecure people who lack confidence in their abilities. They may seek to protect themselves emotionally, and for this reason often appear selfish. Because of their personality traits, neurotic people frequently experience difficulties in their relationships with colleagues, friends and relatives. Difficult personal relationships only help to make matters worse and produce further problems.

THE CAUSES OF NEUROTIC ILLNESS

Under stress, the person with neurotic traits may break down with mental illness. Exactly why this should happen is not known. There is some evidence that the tendency to breakdown may be inherited, but this is doubtful. It is more likely that the cause lies in the upbringing of the child. Over-protective parents may produce a weak and dependent person who is unable to cope with life in an adult way.

It is possible that a neurotic parent can, by example, teach a child to react to problems with neurotic behaviour. There seems little doubt that some neurotic behaviour is learned in this way.

The neuroses are classified as follows:

> Anxiety neurosis
> Phobic anxiety
> Hysteria
> Obsessive-compulsive neurosis
> Reactive depression

ANXIETY NEUROSIS

Anxiety or worry is a common condition experienced by everyone at one time or another. A certain amount of anxiety is expected in everyday life and is considered normal. Indeed, a little anxiety can help a person to overcome difficulties and achieve success. Anxiety is only considered to be an illness when it occurs without a reasonable cause, or when it remains long after the cause has been forgotten.

Causes

Some people are more prone to anxiety than others; the 'born worriers'. Stress situations such as examinations, interviews and difficulties at work will provoke anxiety in those who are prone to it. Less obviously, inner conflicts, e.g. difficult decisions, which often produce feelings of guilt, may create anxiety. The frustration of continued failure may well produce anxiety in those people who can never give up.

Signs and symptoms

The effects of anxiety are both physical and mental. The physical responses are the effects of fear upon the body. Anxiety stimulates the **Adrenal glands** (one situated on top of each kidney) to produce the hormone **Adrenaline**. This hormone prepares the body for any physical emergency, the so-called 'fight or flight' reaction. The important effects of adrenaline on the body, and therefore the physical effects of anxiety, are:

> palpitation of the heart
> increased respiration
> dilatation of the pupils
> sweating
> pallor
> dryness of the mouth
> frequency of micturition
> diarrhoea

Anxious patients experience many of these symptoms and often become afraid of them. Many fear the palpitations and increased respiration to be signs of heart failure, or feel that they are about to choke to death. A severe attack of anxiety with a feeling of impending death is called a **panic attack**.

More often the symptoms are less severe, although they will still worry the patient greatly. Some anxious patients are concerned only with their physical health, demanding repeated examinations and investigations. Such patients are considered **hypochondriacal**.

The anxious person will feel tense and be unable to relax. He may complain of having 'butterflies in the stomach' and weakness of the limbs. In addition he will be constantly worried, unable to concentrate and find great difficulty in getting to sleep (**insomnia**).

Most of the patients admitted to hospital for treatment have no idea of the cause of their anxiety. Many have been anxious and unhappy for months or even years, and are said to be suffering from **chronic** (long-term) anxiety.

Treatment

Only patients who are very anxious will need to be admitted to hospital for treatment. Less anxious people are best treated as out-patients or at home. Some may benefit from a rest and a change of environment, while others are better off remaining at work.

An attack of acute anxiety, if it is severe, may require heavy sedation. In all cases it is important to assure the patient that he is not physically ill. A simple explanation of the physical effects of anxiety will do much to reassure the average person. If the anxiety has an obvious cause, discussion with the nursing and medical staff will often have a calming effect on the patient.

Generally, the anxious patient will be prescribed a mild tranquillizing drug (e.g. Diazepam 5–20 mg three times daily) and a hypnotic at night (e.g. Nitrazepam 5–10 mg). Psychotherapy is often used to help the patient deal with his anxiety and to encourage a more helpful attitude to the problem.

General management

Admission to a psychiatric ward is in itself anxiety-provoking. Every attempt should be made to lessen the patient's immediate worries by introducing him to other patients and staff, and by explaining fully the geography and facilities of the ward.

For many patients, admission to a psychiatric ward confirms their fears of insanity. Anxious patients need reassurance about their mental as well as their physical health, and the nurse can say truthfully that anxiety is not insanity.

The anxious, tense patient will benefit from having something to do while in hospital. If occupational therapy is available so much the better, but the patient can be occupied on the ward by providing him with small tasks helpful to ward routine.

The outlook for the patient suffering from acute anxiety is good. However, chronic anxiety states tend to persist, although the patient can be helped with tranquillizers and continued support from nurses, doctors and social workers.

PHOBIC ANXIETY

A phobia is an unreasonable fear of an object or situation. The phobic patient will be terrified when confronted with the situation he dislikes, and the symptoms will be similar to those of an acute attack of anxiety (see p. 58). Phobias may include any number of situations. Common objects of phobic anxiety are:

enclosed spaces	**claustrophobia**
open spaces	**agoraphobia**
heights	**acrophobia**
dirt	**mysophobia**
dogs	**cynophobia**
travelling	**hodophobia**

It is thought that phobias occur only in people who are prone to anxiety. If this is true, then the phobia only hides the real cause of the patient's worries. On the other hand, it is well known that fears can be passed on from one person to another, particularly from parent to child. The mother who is terrified of mice will no doubt teach her daughter to be frightened of mice also.

Whatever the cause of phobic anxiety, the illness can bring great misery to those who suffer from it. If the fear extends into everyday situations the condition can be crippling. A fear of travelling (and this is quite common) will mean that the patient is restricted to his neighbourhood. Agoraphobia often means that the patient is entirely housebound, and much publicity has recently been given to the plight of countless housewives who have not left their homes for several years.

Phobic anxiety will often be relieved by psychotherapy and, in some cases, minor tranquillizers. The treatment commonly used for phobic anxiety is desensitisation therapy (see 178).

HYSTERIA

In this type of neurosis the patient displays physical and mental signs in order to avoid anxious situations or gain some personal end. Hysterical behaviour can be very frightening to onlookers, although the reasons for it are sometimes obvious. Hysterics are openly indifferent to the effects of their behaviour on others, and this can annoy relatives and people in close contact with them. Eventually the patient may be regarded as a malingerer.

Hysterical patients express their anxiety physically in the form of paralysis, blindness, deafness, fainting, vomiting and epileptiform fits. They may also produce mental symptoms such as **amnesia** (loss of memory) and **fugues** (wandering away and being unable to give an explanation). The symptoms are produced unconsciously, but always serve a purpose for the patient. For example, a student who is afraid to sit his examinations may develop a paralysed hand, while the man who is unhappily married may develop amnesia for a time after his marriage.

Although it may be easy for us to see the reasons for hysterical behaviour, the patient certainly cannot. The hysteric has no control over the production of his symptoms, unlike a malingerer who can suddenly develop a 'headache'. The symptoms have no physical cause, yet they are very real to the patient. A hysterical paralysis of the hand is a real paralysis to the patient; he simply cannot move his hand.

Hysterical people often possess personalities which arouse anger in others. They can be insincere, theatrical types, over-emotional and dramatic. Nurses may find it difficult to feel sympathetic towards them, but it is important to remember always that the hysterical patient is suffering from a very real mental illness.

The treatment which holds the most hope for hysterical patients is psychotherapy (see p. 175). It is important to get the patient to see for himself the reasons for his behaviour, but this is difficult. It is often questioned by nurses whether it is right to give attention to patients who are behaving in a hysterical way. Pandering to the patient who is behaving hysterically is likely only to produce more symptoms. However, hysterical patients when behaving reasonably should not be ignored. In this way, it is possible to teach the patient that attention can only be gained by responsible, adult behaviour.

OBSESSIVE—COMPULSIVE NEUROSIS

In this condition the patient is compelled to constantly repeat certain thoughts or actions, much against his wish. The inner force which compels him is anxiety, and it becomes too great to bear if he tries to ignore his feelings. The illness is most distressing for the patient because he realises that his behaviour is abnormal, and yet he can do nothing about it. Obsessional people are often hard-working individuals, but with a rigid attitude to life that makes it almost impossible for them to relax.

Obsessions are thoughts and ideas which force themselves into the person's mind against his wish. Any attempt to stop them produces anxiety and their return to the mind. Obsessions can range over a variety of subjects. Ideas of doubt are common; for example, the patient doubting whether he has turned off the gas taps or locked the doors at night. Sometimes he may think about an object or word for a long time, asking himself numerous questions about it. Obsessional patients can become so pre-occupied that they are unable to think about the concerns of everyday life.

A **compulsion** is an irresistible urge from within, which forces the person to perform certain acts. Compulsions often follow from obsessional thoughts. The patient who doubts whether he has locked the door may be compelled to go repeatedly to check. Often the checking has to be repeated a certain number of times, the actual number having a 'magical' meaning for the patient. Other compulsions involve washing repeatedly, touching things and moving things from place to place. Any attempt by the patient to ignore the compulsion creates great anxiety in him and a feeling that something bad will happen.

Obsessional fears produce great anxiety and are often seen in phobic anxiety (see p. 60). Fears of dirt, bacteria and contamination are common and may lead the patient to avoid touching certain objects or people. Some patients have a complicated list of things they must avoid, and in such cases life can become unbearable. Others wash so much that their hands become raw with constant scrubbing. Boiling cutlery, constantly changing linen and clothes, sweeping and washing objects with disinfectant are all further examples of obsessional behaviour.

Treatment

The treatments for obsessive–compulsive neurosis are not always successful. Many patients are admitted to hospital exhausted and depressed by the illness. Anti-depressant, sedative and tranquillizing drugs help the patient to some extent, but do little to overcome the obsessions. Psychotherapy and behaviour therapy are useful for these patients, and in selected cases Anafranil Infusion Therapy (see p. 183) can be of benefit.

Obsessive–compulsive neurosis is seldom seen in people over the age of forty years. In those cases where treatment has been unsuccessful, there is some hope that the symptoms will become less severe with advancing age.

REACTIVE DEPRESSION

Reactive Depression means depression of mood as a result of unfortunate circumstances. The causes of this illness are numerous. It can occur after bereavements, broken love affairs, unemployment or failure. Depression may also result from personality difficulties which produce unsatisfactory relationships with others, or involve feelings of guilt.

Everyone has been at least mildly depressed at some time, and so the feelings of the patient suffering from reactive depression are easily understood. Although the depression is not as severe as the depression seen in psychotic illness (see Chapter 7) the patient's mood may be very low. He will often complain of headache, insomnia and tiredness. His appetite will be poor and he will spend a great deal of time thinking about his problems. In a few cases suicidal attempts may be made, but they are not generally serious. However, a few reactive depressives have succeeded in ending their lives, and all suicidal gestures must be taken seriously (see p. 164).

The patient suffering from reactive depression will want to talk about his problems, and will gain great benefit from being allowed to do so. He should be encouraged to see his problems in perspective and given much support. Drug therapy may include the use of antidepressants and mild tranquillizers, but these will be used carefully by the medical staff because of the risk that the patient may come to depend on them.

There is no reason why the patient suffering from reactive depression should not recover completely once his problems diminish or he is helped to deal with them. Even those people who become depressed after minor setbacks and misfortunes can be helped with continued support and advice.

CASE ILLUSTRATION 1: ANXIETY NEUROSIS

Mrs Roberts was in tears as she entered the charge nurse's office. 'Will he ever get better? He was so worried when he came here, but now he seems to have got worse. Have you seen him? He has been mumbling all the time I've been here, and I can't understand what he is saying. Nothing I can do will make him sit still for a moment.'

'Now come and sit down Mrs Roberts. I'll find your husband and see if there is anything I can do. I'm sure he is going to be all right.' The charge nurse left the office and walked into the dormitory where he knew Mr Roberts would be. When he arrived Mr Roberts was on his hands and knees beside his bed, picking fluff from the carpet and collecting it in his hands. 'Mr Roberts, come and lie on your bed for a while.' He helped him to his feet, and Mr Roberts sat on the edge of his bed, trembling. The charge nurse checked his pulse and respiration; both were raised. Sweat was pouring from his face, and he looked pale and drawn.

Jack Roberts had been admitted to hospital two weeks ago. A milkman for almost twenty years, he had recently been offered the job of assistant manager at the dairy. He was reluctant to take the job at first, but at his wife's insistence he eventually accepted. A few weeks after starting his new job he began to get dizzy spells, accompanied by blurred vision. Although the attacks came at any time, they were more frequent while he was at work. He found it increasingly difficult to add up the figures which were an important part of his work. He began to suffer from shortness of breath, and at times this would become so bad that he would have to leave the office and go outside for air. At first he thought that this must be because he had worked for so long in the open air, but later decided that he must be physically ill. Mr Roberts went to see his G.P., who sent him along to the cardiology department of the local general hospital. Investigations there revealed that there was nothing physically wrong, and at last his doctor made an appointment for him at the psychiatric out-patients clinic. The doctor who examined him at the clinic advised a short period of treatment in hospital. Until now everyone had been pleased with Jack's progress, especially his wife who was looking forward to his return home.

Before returning to speak with Mrs Roberts, the charge nurse asked the staff nurse to give Mr Roberts the intra-muscular injection of diazepam, which had been prescribed for such an emergency. On his return to the office he found Mrs Roberts very upset. 'Now don't worry Mrs Roberts, I have given your husband something which will make him feel better. Did you speak to him today about his discharge from hospital?' 'Well, yes I did', replied Mrs Roberts. 'He seemed so well yesterday that I thought it would not be long before he could come home. I told him that I went to see the manager of the dairy, and that he was looking forward to having him back at work.' 'I think that it may be a good idea not to talk about his discharge when you visit him tomorrow,' said the charge nurse. 'He is getting better, but he is not well enough yet to want to talk about these things.'

Mr Roberts remained in hospital for a further five weeks. His wife took the advice of the charge nurse, and he maintained good improvement. He continued to take 10 mg of diazepam three times daily, and this was reduced to 5 mg three times daily during the final week of his stay. During the last few nights in hospital he declined to take his night sedation, stating that he could sleep well enough without it.

At one of the group therapy sessions, which Mr Roberts attended regularly, he said that he would be very happy if he could go back to his previous job as a milkman. After a discussion with the doctor, Mrs Roberts agreed that this would be better for her husband, although she was disappointed.

Mr Roberts was discharged home into the care of his family

doctor. He was asked to continue with diazepam 5 mg three times a day, but told that he could omit the lunch time dose if he began to feel tired. He returned to his previous employment as a milkman.

CASE ILLUSTRATION 2:
PHOBIC ANXIETY – agoraphobia

'I don't know why it is, doctor,' said Mrs Reynolds who was sitting nervously in the chair. 'It started a year ago. I shall always remember it. The bus was very crowded, and held up in a traffic jam in the centre of town. It seemed as if the journey to work would never end. Suddenly the people on the bus seemed to get bigger and bigger, and then the whole bus closed in on me; I thought I was going to suffocate. I woke up in a shop; the sales girl was very kind. She got the van driver to take me straight home. I really felt awful. Soon after, it happened again in the supermarket. I felt that I was going to die, and I just left the shopping and ran home. Then it began to happen in the street, every time I went out. In the end I was too afraid to go out at all.'

'How long is it since you have been out, Mrs Reynolds?' asked the doctor. 'It must be four months at least, until this morning of course.' 'And how did you get to the hospital this morning?' 'My husband drove me here.' 'Did you feel nervous on the way here?' 'Yes, terribly – I feel sorry for my husband. He has taken the day off work to drive me here, and we can't really afford it. I have had to give up work, and we have a lot of expense, what with the mortgage and everything.' 'How many children have you got, Mrs Reynolds?' 'Two, doctor, and I feel awful when I think of how they are neglected.' 'Neglected, what do you mean?' 'Well, yes, I can't take them out, I can't go to the shops to buy their food – my husband goes to the shops at week-ends.' 'But you manage to cook for them.' 'Oh yes, I feel perfectly all right at home. The children are very good. The eldest looks after her young brother, takes him to school before she gets on the bus to her own school, and takes him to the park at week-ends.'

The doctor took another look at the social worker's report in front of him, to refresh his memory. This patient has a nice home, and her children are well cared for. She became pregnant eighteen months ago, and requested an abortion because she felt too nervous to go through with another pregnancy and care for a young baby. After the abortion she became depressed, although this is not unnatural. She does not like to talk about her abortion, but she obviously thinks about it a lot.

The doctor looked up and spoke to Mrs Reynolds. 'Now Mrs Reynolds, I am going to try to help you overcome this fear of going out. I am going to arrange for you to come to the occupational therapy centre each week from Monday to Friday. There will be other people to talk with there, and people who will help you. You need not worry, I will arrange for an ambulance to collect you from home each morning and take you back in the afternoon. I go to the occupational therapy centre two days a week, and you will find that I and all the other patients have a meeting then. I would like you to join us at those meetings. In the meantime I want you to take one of these tablets three times a day.' The doctor began to write a prescription for lorazepam. 'Will I be all right doctor? I will eventually be able to go out won't I?' 'Well, Mrs Reynolds, we have patients who were indoors for ten years or longer, and many of them are able to go to work now.'

Mrs Reynolds attended the occupational therapy centre for ten months. At first she was anxious about making the journey to hospital by ambulance each day, but soon came to know the ambulance men and feel more at ease. At the centre she learned typing, as this was something she always wanted to do. She became quite proud of her progress, and worked constantly towards improving her speed.

After a few weeks, it was decided to ask the community nursing officer if he could arrange for a nurse to visit Mrs Reynolds at home and take her out for short walks. She had already started to take walks with the other patients in the hospital grounds, and felt quite at ease in doing so. A community nurse came to see Mrs Reynolds in the centre to explain what she hoped to do. Mrs Reynolds seemed quite pleased, and took to her instantly.

The visits were arranged for Saturday mornings. At first the nurse would accompany Mrs Reynolds for short walks down the street, and later across the busy main road. After several weeks Mrs Reynolds built up enough courage to get on to a bus with the nurse to go to the local shops. The week-end bus rides to the shops became regular features, and almost without realising it Mrs Reynolds came to look forward to the outings.

It was a fine sunny morning when Mrs Reynolds said goodbye to her husband and children, and started to change for her journey to the hospital. The ambulance would arrive very soon. Suddenly she thought 'What would they say at the hospital if I went there by bus, on my own?' She hurriedly dressed, collected her purse and handbag, and closed the door behind her. On the bus she sat in the seat nearest the door. 'What happens if I have to get off now?' she thought. 'The ambulance must have left without me a long time ago.'

When she walked into the centre, at least thirty minutes late, she was greeted by the typing instructor. 'Whatever happened, Mrs Reynolds? We thought you weren't coming today.' She could hardly control her voice when she answered, 'I don't think I need that ambulance again, can you cancel it?'

CASE ILLUSTRATION 3:
OBSESSIVE–COMPULSIVE NEUROSIS

'I'm Mrs Swift,' said the neatly dressed lady in her early 30s, 'I've come to see Dr Rogers.' 'Yes of course,' replied the nurse extending her hand, 'we are expecting you.' 'I'm sorry, but I can't shake hands with you,' said Mrs Swift apologetically, 'you see, I'll have to wash them again if I do. I'm so sorry, it's so embarrassing. I don't mean to offend you.' The nurse withdrew her hand and escorted Mrs Swift into the empty waiting room. 'Please sit down Mrs Swift, I'll see if Dr Rogers can see you now.'

'I'm sorry Mrs Swift,' said the nurse when she returned a few minutes later, 'Dr Rogers is busy just now, but he will be able to see you in twenty minutes or so. Why don't you sit down and wait?' 'No thank you nurse, I really can't.' 'Why not?' the nurse asked. 'Well, if I sit down I will have to take these clothes to the cleaner's when I get home, and I don't really have anything else to wear. I have other clothes of course, but they are all at the cleaner's.' 'Why, Mrs Swift?' asked the nurse, as she sat on the arm of the chair. 'I don't know really, it's just that when I sit in a chair that doesn't belong to me I have to take my clothes to the cleaner's afterwards.' 'Would you like a cup of tea, Mrs Swift? I'll bring a cup for you to drink while you're waiting.'

The nurse returned a few minutes later with two cups of tea on a tray. 'Sugar, Mrs Swift?' she said, offering her the sugar bowl. Mrs Swift picked up a teaspoon of sugar, and for a few seconds moved it back and forth over the cup and sugar bowl. 'Do you generally take sugar, Mrs Swift?' asked the nurse. 'Yes I do, but . . .' The nurse took the spoon from Mrs Swift and put sugar into her cup. She glanced at the cup, then at the sugar bowl and finally at the nurse. 'I couldn't decide you see.'

'How long have you been feeling anxious?' asked the nurse. She knew that it must have been for some time, as the patient looked so pale and drawn. 'Ten years or so, but it seems to have got worse lately.' Mrs Swift obviously wanted to talk about her problem, and so the nurse listened. 'My husband is just about fed up with everything, not that I blame him. You see, I have to do silly things all the time.' 'What sort of silly things?' asked the nurse. 'Well, everything has to be in order before I go to bed. It takes me more than an hour to get to sleep because I have to go around the house checking all the taps and doors. I have to go back and check seven times. If I don't do it I can't get to sleep for worry. Then in the morning, after I've prepared breakfast, the washing-up takes such a long time. Everything has to be rinsed in hot water seven times. Then I have to swab the draining-board with disinfectant and pour boiling water over it.'

'Do you cook meals for your husband, Mrs Swift?' 'Yes, some-times I do. You see, everything takes such a long time that I have to choose between the housework or cooking a meal. It takes all day to do either. Yesterday it took me an hour to place the clock in the right position on the sideboard. I kept thinking that it must be exactly level you see. Sometimes it takes me half an hour to go from one room to another. I have to keep going back to see if the door is closed, and to touch the door knob.' 'Have you tried not doing all these things, Mrs Swift? You did say they were silly.' 'I have tried, but the worry is too great to bear. I keep thinking that my husband will die or meet with an accident, or that my children will die if I don't do these things. My poor children, I can't even cook for them.' 'How do you manage with the children, Mrs Swift?' 'My sister comes in every day to take care of them, and they both go to school of course. My mother has offered to help, but you see she has the same problem, but she isn't quite so bad as I am.'

After his interview with Mrs Swift the doctor decided that she should be admitted to hospital. She had reached the point of exhaustion, and although she did not mention it to the nurse, she was contemplating suicide. She was admitted that afternoon, and was prescribed tranquillizing drugs and nightly sedation. When her physical condition improved, she started to attend regular psychotherapy sessions on an individual basis. Three months later she had at least recovered sufficiently to be able to cope with her rituals at home, without placing too much stress on the rest of her family.

CASE ILLUSTRATION 4: HYSTERIA

George Black looked miserable as he walked into the doctor's office for one of his regular interviews. 'How are you today?' asked the doctor. 'I'm not feeling well doctor,' answered George sadly. 'I'm worried about my wife and children. Nothing is being done for them. They have no electricity, no gas, and it's so cold. I don't know what I'm going to do. I cry when I go home to see them. I can't do anything; my arm, you see.' 'How is your arm today?' George's right arm hung limply at his side as he sat in the chair. 'I still can't move it, doctor. You can't do anything, can you? The nurses aren't helping me either. They won't even cut my food up for me. It's difficult to eat with one arm you know. They are wicked, it just isn't fair. I've always been kind to people.' 'Perhaps you would like to go home for a few days to see what you can do for your wife, George,' said the doctor, knowing what the answer would be. 'How can I go home like this?' 'Look George', said the doctor, 'we are all trying to help you. The nurses probably think that you should try to use your arm to get it moving again. You see my leg' – the doctor pointed to his right leg which had been injured in an accident a few weeeks ago – 'I have to exercise it or I will always have this limp.' 'They are just being wicked,' said George. No amount of persuasion would convince George that he did not have a physical disease. The doctor had tried so many times, in so many different ways before.

George had a strange effect on the nursing staff, but it was an effect they all recognised and knew how to handle. A little man, George was always polite, and willing to help with the ward work despite his 'paralysis'. In fact, he gave an impression of being a martyr, always saying how hard he worked while the other patients, with all four limbs, did nothing. This was the annoying effect George had. The fact that he would not – or so far as he was concerned, could not – help himself, added to the annoyance.

But still, one could not help feeling sorry for George. He had worked in a factory for seven years, saving hard to buy a small newsagent's shop. Eighteen months ago he bought his shop, but was, as he put it, 'taken for a ride'. The shop was situated near another newsagent's, and a street news seller had set up a stand just round the corner. The business was in decline when George bought it, although he was not aware of this. Within a few months he was in debt, and eventually bankruptcy proceedings were taken against him. The shop was closed, but he was allowed to remain in the accommodation above. The gas and electricity bills could not be paid, and the supplies were cut off. Soon after the bankruptcy hearing was over, George found that he was unable to move his right arm.

After his admission to hospital, the social worker made many appeals to the Gas and Electricity Boards to restore supplies. They refused because George was legally bankrupt, and had no means of paying his debts. George could not be persuaded to start work in a factory again; the only thing he could do if things were to be improved. He wanted help. Help from the doctor, the social services, the Department of Health and Social Security, in fact anyone who would give it. His paralysis must surely produce some sympathy.

It was a week later, when George had returned from a visit home, that he demanded to see the doctor again. He waited at the door of the ward for his arrival. The doctor eventually came, and limped along the corridor. George walked beside him, and had already started to talk about his problems when the doctor noticed something strange. George had developed a limp in his right leg.

George Black remained in hospital for almost a year. He attended group therapy sessions for all of that time. Slowly he began to realise that his problems, instead of getting better as he had hoped, were gradually getting worse. His paralysis eventually improved, and despite several relapses, vanished completely after some months. He is once again working in a local factory.

CASE ILLUSTRATION 5: REACTIVE DEPRESSION

John Potter looked, and indeed felt, very depressed. He sat in an armchair hour after hour, only getting up for meals. In the evenings he went to the lounge to watch television. Not that he was interested in food or television, but somehow he felt that he had to make an effort. He was never very hungry, and picked at his food, leaving much of it on the plate. Television was dull, and besides he found it very hard to concentrate. He was constantly worried, and thinking what he was going to do now that he was alone. After all, he was nearly fifty. The idea of going home to an empty house filled him with fear, and so for that matter did the thought of returning to work.

Only the nurses provided some comfort for John Potter in that ward. He could talk to them, and they were always willing to listen. Of course, they couldn't do very much for him. Neither could the doctor, or anyone else for that matter. He was going to be miserable for the rest of his life. She would be sorry if he did kill himself in the end, of that he was certain. If only she knew how he was suffering, she would come back. If she didn't, then it was his greatest misfortune to have married someone like her in the first place. Deceptive; he knew all along how deceptive she could be.

It was after a hard day's work that John Potter came home to find that his wife and children had gone. She had left a letter giving her address. She had gone to stay with her brother and his wife in Wales. 'You can write if you wish,' she had said, 'but please don't come to see me.' Why has she done this? There was no other man so far as he knew. He had provided a nice home; they were comfortably off. He was quite happy, and assumed that she was too. Yes, he worked long hours, but he had explained why and she seemed not to mind.

The very next day John Potter drove to Wales. His brother-in-law answered the door of the small house where his wife was staying, but refused to let him in. Two weeks later he received a letter from his wife's solicitor informing him that divorce proceedings would be started in the near future.

John became more and more miserable. One night, in deep despair, he decided that he might be better off dead. He wrote a letter to his wife, and swallowed the remaining sleeping pills in the bottle he had got from his doctor.

John awoke in the ward of a general hospital. At first he was relieved that someone had found him, and that he was still alive, but his misery soon returned. A doctor from the local psychiatric hospital came to see him, and it was on his advice that he was eventually admitted there.

John remained in hospital for six weeks. After a short time he began to improve and took a little interest in his surroundings. He started to attend the ward meetings, and was later offered a place in the woodwork department of the occupational therapy centre. John liked woodwork, and it had the effect of taking his mind off his worries for at least a few hours a day. The tranquillizing drugs which the doctor prescribed helped him too, and he found that he was beginning to worry less as time passed.

A week before he left hospital John received a letter from his wife, asking if she might come to visit him. Whatever might happen in the future, John was more confident that he would be able to deal with his problems.

QUESTIONS

1   Name three types of neurotic illness.

*2 Name two symptoms arising from anxiety.

3 What do you understand by the term 'panic attack'?

4 What is meant by the term 'phobia'?

5 Name two treatments for phobic anxiety.

6 State three personality characteristics sometimes found in hysterical patients.

7 What do you understand by the term 'obsession'?

8 Give one example of an obsession.

9 Give one example of a compulsion.

10 Name two treatments for obsessive–compulsive neurosis.

11 What do you understand by the term 'reactive depression'?

12 What do you understand by the term 'neurosis'?

* Reproduced by permission of The General Nursing Council for England and Wales.

Chapter 7

FUNCTIONAL PSYCHOSES

The psychoses are a group of severe mental illnesses which give rise to marked changes in the patient's personality and behaviour. Generally psychotic patients do not fully realise that they are ill, and we say that they **lack insight** into their illness.

The word **functional** when used to describe a mental illness means without physical cause, and the functional psychoses are those which do not have any known physical cause. There are three functional psychoses, Manic-depressive Psychosis, Involutional Melancholia and Schizophrenia.

MANIC-DEPRESSIVE PSYCHOSIS

Manic-depressive Psychosis is basically a disorder of mood. In this illness the patient will either become very depressed or abnormally happy and energetic. Very occasionally a patient will experience both extremes, his mood alternating quite quickly from elation to depression. Usually however, these patients suffer from only one abnormal mood without ever experiencing the other. These disorders of mood are discussed separately under the headings of Mania and Endogenous Depression.

MANIA

Mania is the name given to the part of the illness when the patient is excessively happy and energetic. In very severe cases the manic patient may become angry and destructive, but this does not often happen. More usually these patients are admitted to hospital in a mildly excited state which we call **hypomania** (hypo = below).

The hypomanic patient will talk a great deal, often in a loud voice and sometimes about personal and embarrassing subjects. He will like nothing better than to involve himself in conversation with others, forcefully stating his point of view. Because of his excessive energy, the hypomanic will be seen dusting, sweeping and re-arranging, or simply interfering in the affairs of others, giving a none too helping hand. This abnormally energetic behaviour is called **overactivity**.

The hypomanic patient is easily distracted by new ideas and situations, and he will seldom finish one task before undertaking the next. Because of his overactivity he will find difficulty in sleeping, and even eating may be overlooked as newer and more exciting ventures attract his attention. The restraint which we practice from day to day is diminished in hypomania, and so the patient may swear, steal, spend all his money or make sexual advances without shame.

It is readily seen that the hypomanic patient will be admitted to hospital when his behaviour eventually tires his relatives and friends. Even in hospital, his initially amusing behaviour will quickly annoy other patients, and it is not unusual to find the hypomanic at the centre of any argument or disturbance in the ward.

If the patient's overactivity increases he will eventually reach the full **manic state**. In this state he will be extremely excited, and may dance, shout and sing at the top of his voice. At this stage delusions of grandeur may develop (see p. 43). and he may become argumentative and aggressive.

Treatment
Drug therapy is the most usual treatment for mania and hypomania. Sedatives (e.g. Sodium Amylobarbitone 200–400 mg) are used to control excited behaviour and to help the patient to sleep. The major tranquillizers (e.g. Chlorpromazine, Triflu-operazine, Haloperidol) are prescribed to help lower the patient's mood and control his behaviour. Lithium Carbonate is another drug which may be used to calm the overactive patient. Group psychotherapy is useful in controlling behaviour, but only when the patient is calm enough to engage in reasonable conversation.

General management
In the hospital ward the overactive patient is best managed by

providing him with occupation that will use up his energy without exciting him. The choice of occupation depends upon the level of his activity and, of course, the type of work available. A job which involves physical activity is best; such as sweeping, polishing and washing up. If the ward has a garden, then supervised work outside is ideal.

If the patient has to be discouraged from doing things which interfere with or annoy others, it is best to try to distract him by suggesting other more suitable activities. Giving the patient his own way over small matters is a good idea if it avoids argument and ill-feeling. In severe cases, where violent behaviour occurs, several nurses must deal with the patient in a firm but sympathetic manner. (The problem of violent behaviour is dealt with in Chapter 14.)

The most important aspect of physical care is to ensure that the patient takes adequate food and fluid. If he is very excited he may not have time to eat a meal, but sandwiches and drinks handed to him will be taken while he continues his activities. Washing and bathing will need to be supervised as the patient may well neglect his personal hygiene.

With modern drug treatments the outlook for the hypomanic or manic patient is very good. The length of stay in hospital depends upon the patient's response to treatment, but there is no reason why he should not return home within a reasonable period of time.

ENDOGENOUS DEPRESSION

Endogenous means from within, and endogenous depression is depression which can develop without an outside cause. It is the depressive phase of manic-depressive psychosis, but may occur in patients who never become manic.

The depressed patient feels and behaves in a way exactly opposite to the manic patient. His mood will be low and he will lose interest in events and his surroundings, sometimes to the extent of not talking at all to other people. He may become so lacking in energy that he will want to sit down all day, finding it an effort even to move from one chair to another. Even thinking may be slow and painful for the depressed person, and even then his thoughts will be miserable and unpleasant. Such patients look, and feel despondent. Their sad, fixed expression, pale, cold skin, paint a very real picture of their inner feelings.

Depressed patients often find difficulty in sleeping, and may wake in the early hours when they feel at their very worst. Eating may become impossible, not only because appetite is lost, but because of the effort involved in feeding. Many of them are troubled by severe, constant headache.

Severely depressed patients may become deluded, believing that they have no money or that they have a dreadful, incurable disease. Some may even believe that they are so wicked that they should be in Hell (see delusions, p. 44).

Suicide is a very real danger in endogenous depression. The patient may feel so miserable and hopeless that death seems the only possible way out for him. The danger of suicide is greatest in patients who are deluded or troubled by constant headache. All depressed patients must be carefully observed, but where there is a very real danger of suicide, the special precautions against suicide must be strictly enforced (see p. 64).

Not all depressed patients are so worn down by their illness that they sit silently for hours. Some patients are only mildly depressed, and manage to remain active and even continue at work. A few remain active even though their mood may be very low indeed, and try hard to hide their true feelings. Such patients may be seriously thinking of suicide without the knowledge of others.

Treatment

With modern treatment endogenous depression can be relieved in a few weeks. Electro-convulsive Therapy (E.C.T.) (see p. 185) is widely used in combination with antidepressant drugs. Sometimes only drugs are used to treat this depression, and examples of these drugs are Amitriptyline, Imipramine or the Monoamine Oxidase Inhibitor drugs (e.g. Marplan, Parnate) (see p. 183).

Psychotherapy is useful to the depressed patient when he has recovered sufficiently to take an interest in his surroundings, and occupational therapy is a necessary part of the treatment of all depressive illnesses.

INVOLUTIONAL MELANCHOLIA

Melancholia is another name for depression and Involutional Melancholia is depression which occurs for the first time in middle age – the involutional period of life.

This illness is very similar to endogenous depression. The patients who suffer from it often show an excessive concern for bodily functions, they may believe that their bowels are blocked, or that they have some terrible disease such as cancer or syphilis. Commonly they accuse themselves of wickedness or sin, and may even come to believe that they are in Hell.

As with endogenous depression, the risk of suicide is always present in involutional melancholia. Problems may arise if the patient refuses to eat, and in these cases the doctor may authorise tube feeding. The treatment with antidepressant drugs and Electro-convulsive Therapy is similar to the treatment of endogenous depression.

SCHIZOPHRENIA

The word **schizophrenia** means 'split mind'. It is a misleading name for the illness, because 'split mind' implies that the sufferer has a good and an evil personality which alternate at a moment's notice. It is also unfortunate that, in the eyes of the public, schizophrenia has become associated with violent murders and other serious crimes. Most schizophrenics do not commit criminal acts. Neither do they have a 'split personality' as so many people believe. Schizophrenia is a severe mental illness which can destroy the personality, leaving the patient unable to deal with even the most simple aspects of daily living.

The effect of schizophrenia is to so alter the patient's thinking and perception that he no longer sees the world as we see it. Buildings and people may take on a different appearance, the things other people say and do take on a different meaning, and even the patient himself may feel changed in some way. For example, one schizophrenic, passing a group of children in a school playground, saw only a stone building with iron bars surrounding it which prevented the children from escaping. He assumed that the children were imprisoned, and as a result wrote a letter of complaint to the school authorities. Another schizophrenic, whenever anyone glanced in his direction, believed that he was being watched by members of a secret organisation determined to kill him. Yet another saw his own reflection in the mirror as a twisted face crawling with worms.

Quite naturally, schizophrenics will behave oddly because of these strange sensations. Some will become very frightened and try to hide, perhaps refusing to go out. Others will become very angry and even violent because of the strange and frightening experiences. A few will be so interested and involved with what is happening that they sit for hours, refusing to talk or involve themselves with others.

Although physicians have been trying for a long time to discover the cause of schizophrenia, a cause is not yet known. We do know that although people of all ages can develop schizophrenia, a large number first do so in adolescence.

Signs and symptoms
One of the most striking effects of schizophrenia is the way in which it alters the patient's way of thinking. We notice this change quite often when a schizophrenic patient talks. He may use words which sound like nonsense to us or talk about things in a way which we cannot quite understand.

Very often schizophrenics seem to be lazy or untidy in appearance. They may not want to get up or take a bath, or perhaps not want to do any work at all. This is because schizophrenia reduces the drive and will power which prompts us to take care of ourselves and take an interest in life. We are generally in control of the things we say and do, but a schizophrenic may feel that he is being controlled by something outside him. Sometimes a schizophrenic will say that he is being controlled by radio or by a hidden machine.

It is sometimes said that schizophrenics cannot laugh at a joke. That is not always true, but very often they will laugh at something that is not funny, or even at something that is really very sad. Conversely, they may become sad or cry about something which would make us laugh. Sometimes schizophrenics seem to be completely lacking in emotion, as those who have been in contact with long-stay schizophrenic patients will know.

Odd movements or peculiar postures are not always seen in schizophrenia, but in some patients they may be very obvious to onlookers. It is not unusual to see schizophrenic patients standing in odd positions, moving their limbs clumsily or adopting strange facial expressions. Sometimes the patient's ability to move at all is lost, and he will lie still in bed or stand motionless in a corner of the room.

Schizophrenic patients are very often hallucinated and deluded. The delusions can be quite fantastic, and may include imaginary plots, torture, or a belief that parts of the body are missing (see Delusions, p. 43).

The hallucinations can affect any of the five senses (see Hallucinations, p. 45) but are most often auditory and visual. It is not uncommon for schizophrenics to hear voices which threaten or laugh at them. The visual hallucinations can be terrifying, and may include visions of rats and snakes, hideous faces and religious figures. Patients may become frightened, angry or excited because of their hallucinations. Frequently a schizophrenic can be seen apparently talking to himself or looking intently at something, but really he is answering the voices he hears or gazing at his visions.

There are four types of schizophrenic illness. These are:

> Simple Schizophrenia
> Catatonic Schizophrenia
> Hebephrenic Schizophrenia
> Paranoid Schizophrenia

Over the past few years it has become less important for psychiatrists to diagnose the different types of schizophrenia, but it will further our knowledge of the illness if we can learn something about them.

SIMPLE SCHIZOPHRENIA

The most important symptom is the patient's loss of interest in his surroundings. He will prefer to lie in bed or sit by himself rather than join in activities and conversation with others. Sometimes a simple schizophrenic will lose interest even in his personal hygiene, and will need to be supervised when bathing and

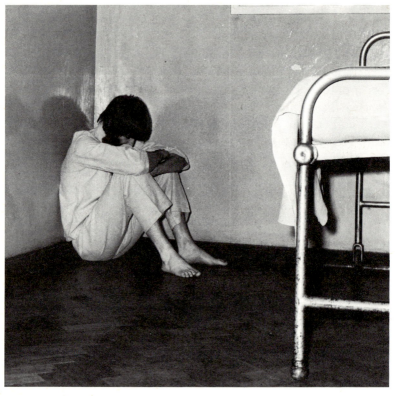

11 The schizophrenic patient can lose contact with the real world

dressing. If he is not encouraged to join in activities, then he will become more and more isolated until it is impossible to communicate with him.

CATATONIC SCHIZOPHRENIA

With this type of schizophrenia the patient will move about in a stiff, clumsy way and hold his limbs in odd, rigid positions. Occasionally a catatonic patient will lie in bed, unable to move or talk, and may appear to be unconscious. This is called a **catatonic**

stupor. Although the patient in a stupor may appear to be unconscious, he is well aware of what is happening around him. When nursing a catatonic patient, care must be taken not to say anything within his hearing that may upset him or make him feel worse. The physical nursing care of a stuporose patient is similar to the care given to a truly unconscious person. The patient's position in bed must be changed every two hours, and an accurate record must be kept of his temperature, pulse and respiration, and of his fluid intake and output. With the aid of modern treatments catatonic stupor seldom continues for long, and tube feeding is hardly ever necessary.

HEBEPHRENIC SCHIZOPHRENIA

This is a very severe type of schizophrenia which occurs in adolescence. The patient will be very disturbed by hallucinations, and may become extremely frightened or aggressive. He will frequently be seen muttering or shouting at his voices. His delusions are often grandiose, and his abnormal thinking may cause him to use words which sound like nonsense. Outbursts of anger or laughter can occur for no apparent reason, and his mood may be quite out of keeping with his thinking and behaviour. Regression is very common, and may be so severe that the patient sits in a corner engrossed with his bizarre thoughts and experiences, neglecting to eat, wash or go to the lavatory.

PARANOID SCHIZOPHRENIA

The paranoid schizophrenic will be very suspicious and troubled by ideas that he is being persecuted. He may believe that others are trying to kill him, that radioactivity is destroying him, or even that others can read his mind. His hallucinations will be very frightening, for he may have visions of devils or wild animals and hear threatening voices.

Paraphrenia and **paranoia** are two other mental illnesses similar to paranoid schizophrenia, which occur in middle age. The paraphrenic patient is more aware of his surroundings than the schizophrenic, in spite of his hallucinations and delusions.

The patient who suffers from paranoia is never hallucinated. His conversation and behaviour may appear so plausible that he is sometimes able to convince other people that his delusions are true.

Not all paranoid patients are aggressive, but even so nursing them can be difficult. A good rule is never to argue with the patient about his delusions, no matter how persistent he may be. Arguing with him is not only useless but will make him more hostile and difficult to manage. The best way to avoid difficulty and help the patient is to accept his ideas calmly without actually agreeing with them. Only with the aid of tact and understanding will the paranoid patient learn to accept and trust the people who are trying to help him.

Treatment

Schizophrenia was at one time an illness from which patients seldom, if ever, recovered. Today, with the help of tranquillizing drugs and other therapeutic methods, the outlook for schizophrenic patients is more hopeful.

As we have seen, schizophrenia is a mental illness which causes the patient to lose contact with the real world and enter a world of imagination and fantasy. The most important aspect of treatment is to encourage the patient to take notice of the real world around him, and in this the nurse has a vital part to play. The nurse should speak to the patient even if he does not answer or appear to understand; help him to participate in group activities; encourage him to make decisions for himself and aid him to care for his appearance. In short, the nurse should confront the patient with the real world wherever possible.

Disturbed behaviour, and even delusions and hallucinations can be reduced by the tranquillizing drugs such as Chlorpromazine, Thioridazine and Trifluoperazine. The amount and type of drug prescribed by the doctor will depend on the patient's condition. Once the newly admitted schizophrenic patient has settled in hospital and his behaviour is better controlled, he will be encouraged to attend an industrial therapy or occupational therapy centre within the hospital. Industrial and occupational therapy help the patient to feel useful, to find new outlets for talent and energy, and encourage him to remain in touch with the real world.

Before he is discharged from hospital, the doctor will need to know something about the patient's home environment and the type of work he is going to do. Social workers can provide this information, and also arrange for regular home visits when the patient has left hospital. Some patients will not be able to return to their regular job, either because they no longer feel able to do it or because they have become unemployed. The employment

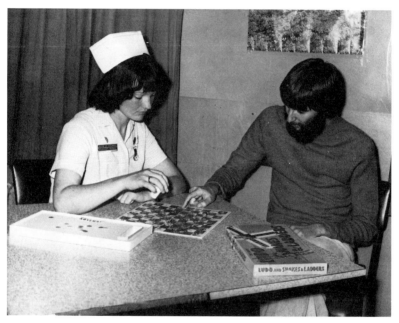

III The nurse should encourage the patient to participate in activities

officer of the hospital can help in finding jobs for patients, while some are encouraged to attend a Government Training Centre where new trades and skills can be learned.

Once the patient is discharged from hospital, every effort will be made to prevent him from returning as an in-patient. Visits to the patient's home by community psychiatric nurses and social workers, and appointments with the psychiatrist can help him to deal with problems without returning to hospital.

The problem of patients not taking their medication regularly is often overcome by the drugs Modecate and Moditen. These are tranquillizers given by intra-muscular injection, either at the patient's home or at hospital, once every two or three weeks (see p. 182).

Even with modern treatments, some schizophrenic patients become ill again and need to be re-admitted to hospital. This should not discourage us in our attempts to help schizophrenics, even if they are admitted time and time again. It is far better for a patient to be admitted to hospital repeatedly than for him to become a permanent resident of a long-stay psychiatric ward.

CASE ILLUSTRATION 6: HYPOMANIA

A small crowd had quickly gathered outside the main post office. Six policemen jumped from the large, black police van and ran inside. Nothing exciting ever happened in this small town, and the arrival of the police in the high street brought shopkeepers and shoppers alike rushing to the scene. The growing crowd moved towards the entrance, as if by some chance they would be able to see through the thick wooden doors the police had shut behind them.

'He won't give me my money,' shouted the small but well-built man to the approaching policemen. 'I have a thousand pounds, and he won't give me a penny of it!' The police sergeant glanced at the counter clerk who was nursing a cut eye, and at the broken glass on the floor. He was in no mood to argue. 'Now just you stop shouting and come with us.' 'I'm not going anywhere, I want my money!' yelled the man. The police moved forward, and with only a slight struggle the man was held on the floor. Two minutes later he was escorted through the crowd outside and into the waiting van.

'Your Worship,' continued the sergeant from the witness box, 'when the clerk refused to give the accused any money, he hit him in the face with his fist, and broke a window with his umbrella.' 'How much money did the accused ask for officer?' asked the magistrate in a sombre tone. 'A thousand pounds,

Your Worship.' The magistrate glanced at the accused who sat
between two policemen, mumbling to himself. 'They are liars!'
the man suddenly screamed, 'I asked for my money, that's all!'
'This is the third time you have interrupted, Mr French,' said the
magistrate severely, 'I will not warn you again. If you shout once
more I shall have you taken to the cells below.' The policeman
finished his evidence, and the magistrate conferred briefly with
the Bench. After a minute or two he spoke to the court. 'We would
like a report on this man from a psychiatrist before we pass
judgement. I am therefore going to adjourn for two weeks so that
a psychiatric report can be obtained.' Looking directly at the
accused he went on, 'Mr French, you will be remanded in custody
for two weeks from today.'

A month later, Peter French was admitted to hospital from the
remand prison. He looked younger than his forty-five years. The
magistrate had decided to order Hospital Treatment under
Section 60 of the Mental Health Act, and so Peter was likely to be
detained for some time. The first thing everyone noticed about
Peter French was his two black eyes, which he said were given
to him in prison because he 'kept singing during the night'.
'How are you, Mr French?' asked the charge nurse, expecting a
hostile reply. 'I'm fine – never felt better,' was the jolly reply.
'Where have the policemen gone? I should have thanked them;
maybe I'll send them a Christmas card. I'd love a drink. Where is
my cell then? I hope it's not pink, I don't like it.' 'Mr French, you
are not in prison now, this is a hospital,' said the charge nurse.
'Hospital, oh, is it? I don't know why I'm in hospital. I had an
operation once. Do you like opera?' and he burst into a badly
sung version of 'Figaro'.

Mr French was still singing as the charge nurse took him upstairs to his side room. 'What a nice place!' he exclaimed, 'I'll
be happy here. I hope the other prisoners are better mannered
than the last lot.' The charge nurse was forced to smile at this
remark. 'I'll have that drink now. "Whisky", I said, didn't I?'
A few minutes later, the charge nurse returned with the
medication which had been prescribed by the doctor. 'I'd like
you to take these tablets Mr French, they will make you feel
better.' 'Of course, old boy,' replied the patient, swallowing the

tablets and the Largactil syrup with relish. 'A good drop of stuff that, but it was a bit strong!'

Peter French soon settled down in hospital. His one complaint was that the 'waiters' did not provide a very good service, but, apart from that, he was no trouble to the nurses. However, several times he got into arguments with the other patients for stealing food and cigarettes from their lockers. At the ward meetings he would say that he particularly liked the way snacks and cigarettes were freely available, to the annoyance of his fellow patients.

As Mr French improved, it was decided to keep him out of mischief by giving him some work to do. He was a hard worker, and in no time had the ward kitchen spotlessly clean, and of course, entirely under his control. The decision was a good one, as he almost never got into trouble while he was working there.

After a month in hospital Mr French had returned to normal. He was able to discuss his problems rationally, and it appeared that just before his breakdown his wife had left him. He recalled feeling miserable for a few days after this event, but could not remember much about the circumstances which led to his appearance in court. He felt rather embarrassed about his behaviour in hospital, and tried to recompense the other patients by buying them cigarettes. He admitted that during the time he was overactive he really felt very miserable.

Peter French remained in hospital for just over six months, and was sent home on extended leave. He is now working, and has not been re-admitted.

CASE ILLUSTRATION 7:
ENDOGENOUS DEPRESSION

'I can't nurse, please, no more,' moaned Colin Bishop as the nurse tried to get another teaspoonful of food into his mouth. 'Well, try a small drink then,' said the nurse, picking up a feeding cup of warm milk. 'No, I can't. Another mouthful will block my throat. I'm full up to here,' the patient pointed to an indefinite area of his chest. 'I haven't been to the lavatory for a week.' 'Well of course not, Mr Bishop,' said the nurse. 'How can you expect to go to the lavatory when you haven't eaten anything?' 'I can't eat. I've told you before, my bowels are blocked up.' 'All right Mr Bishop, but you'll have to try again later.' His eyes followed the nurse as she picked up the dishes and turned away.

It was an ordeal trying to get Colin Bishop to eat. For a week he had eaten only two or three teaspoonfuls a day. Two days ago he began to refuse drinks. Now he remained in bed all day, becoming progressively weaker and starting to dehydrate. Something would have to be done shortly to ensure that he took fluid.

Colin Bishop was a depressive. After six previous admissions to hospital, with the same symptoms, that was a safe enough diagnosis. All his admissions had been preceded by similar events. He would feel tired and miserable, and find it hard to remain asleep for very long. He would start to worry his wife with imaginary financial problems; saying that they were in debt and could not afford to eat such lavish meals. Then he would give up eating almost entirely. From past experience, Mrs Bishop would call in the family doctor, and arrangements would be made for Colin to be admitted to hospital.

To start with, this present depression had begun in the familiar way. As usual, he had been to the bank to order a stop on all cheques drawn on his joint account, leaving his wife without a penny. This time, however, he had told his wife that he had cancer, and that he did not have long to live. This was a new development, and Mrs Bishop began to worry more than usual. Colin was going into hospital, but not for another two days. The day before his admission was due he told his wife that he was going to see his brother to 'make arrangements for the debts to be paid'. Colin was out for a long time, and Mrs Bishop became extremely worried. The telephone rang. He had already been admitted to hospital. He was found standing at the end of the station platform, waiting to jump.

Regarded as a suicidal risk by the nursing and medical staff, Colin was given a bed in the observation dormitory. He was a pitiful sight. Lying in bed he did nothing but wring his hands and moan. 'This is Hell – I must be in Hell.' He would only talk about his cancer and how it was blocking his inside. 'Even if I could eat the food, I couldn't afford to pay,' he would say. 'I want to die, why won't somebody kill me?'

The charge nurse told the doctor about Colin's deteriorating condition. There was not likely to be an improvement, as he refused to take his medication. He was now quite dehydrated, the charge nurse explained. The doctor examined Colin and ordered that he should be tube fed without delay.

The tube feeding was an ordeal for Colin. He did not struggle, but regarded the nurses as people who were there to torture him. After two days of being tube-fed water, Complan and the necessary salt and vitamins, Colin was well enough for his first E.C.T. The consent for the administration of the anaesthetic had already been obtained from his wife, as he was in no position to agree or disagree. When Colin was told that he was to have E.C.T. he replied 'Good, at last you are going to kill me. Get it over with quickly, unless you want me to suffer longer.'

Colin had a course of six E.C.Ts. He began to improve after the second treatment, and within a fortnight was eating without encouragement from the nursing staff. He was still depressed however, and needed close observation. His sleep was still very disturbed, and although he could get to sleep easily he would wake in the early hours. Nevertheless, he progressed rapidly, and soon began to take more interest in his surroundings.

Colin was discharged from hospital after seven weeks. He continued as an outpatient, taking 25 mg of imipramine three times daily. A fortnight after his discharge he returned once again to his job as assistant manager of a local bank.

CASE ILLUSTRATION 8: SCHIZOPHRENIA (i)

'Phillip is not interested in his work. He is the most lethargic pupil in class.' So ended the last primary school report before Phillip left to join the local comprehensive school. His reports from there were bad also, and he soon came to be regarded by the teachers as 'a lazy, unco-operative child'. In fact, Phillip was never unco-operative; he was simply uninterested and lacking in initiative.

Life in the comprehensive school was very difficult for Phillip Turner. Situated in the East End of London, the school had a reputation for its large number of aggressive pupils. Phillip was 'picked on' a great deal. He began to play truant, and would spend the day wandering the streets of the neighbourhood. The headmaster saw Mrs Turner about her son's behaviour on several occasions, but Phillip's behaviour and work did not improve.

Shortly after his fifteenth birthday Phillip left school to work as a cleaner in a local factory. He was not interested in the job, always had to be told what to do, and frequently arrived late. He was dismissed after only three months and never held another job.

Phillip lived in a large terraced house with his mother. He was her only child, and her husband had died when Phillip was three years of age. Mrs Turner was a kind but unintelligent woman, and paid little attention to her son's lethargy. She did not object when Phillip refused to wash, shave and take baths, and never encouraged him to find a job. She called him only once in the mornings, and if Phillip refused to get out of bed, as was usual, she would let him lie there all morning.

Mrs Turner had not been physically well for years. She suffered from a heart condition which she neglected as much as her son's unusual behaviour. One lunch time, Phillip got up to find his mother still in bed, and was unable to wake her. He returned to bed himself, and it was not until the next morning, finding her still in bed, that he decided to stop a passer-by in the street to ask for help. The passer-by knocked at the house next door to call an ambulance, and the neighbour was shocked at Phillip's unkempt appearance. Later that day she telephoned the local social service department, and the same evening a social worker called round to see Phillip.

Phillip was admitted to the psychiatric hospital the day after his mother was taken to the local general hospital. He was extremely dirty, said very little, and showed no interest in his surroundings. He was quite co-operative, and willingly took a bath and changed his clothes when told to do so. After his bath, Phillip was interviewed by a doctor. He answered only when spoken to, but nevertheless was able to give an accurate account of what had happened. He did not enquire about his mother, and said only 'yes' when told that she was recovering. Psychological tests given to Phillip a week later showed that he is slightly below average intelligence, and that his memory is intact.

Phillip has been in hospital for two years now. He still has to be told to wash and shave, and would remain in bed all day unless told to get up. During the day he attends the industrial therapy department, but is accompanied by a nurse to ensure that he arrives and remains at work. He talks very little, and then only to answer direct questions. He has no interest in his future, and never asks about his mother who is now living at home. It is evident that he knows exactly where he is, and is perfectly happy to remain in hospital indefinitely. Asked recently what he was going to do when he left hospital he replied, 'I don't know, I like it here.'

CASE ILLUSTRATION 9: SCHIZOPHRENIA (ii)

David Cook had always been a shy, sensitive young man who preferred his own company to that of others. At school he was studious, and left at the age of sixteen to work for a firm of accountants in London. He made very few friends, and in the evenings and at week-ends spent most of his time at home. David's main hobby was astronomy. As soon as it was dark, he would retire to his bedroom to set up the telescope his father had given him on his sixteenth birthday. Since leaving school he had collected a large number of books, most of them about astronomy. His father, quite unable to understand this technical literature, was nevertheless quite proud that he should take up such an intellectual hobby.

One night, as Mr Cook was passing his son's room on his way to bed, he heard voices coming from inside. He knew that no visitors had called that evening, and so he knocked on the bedroom door. David opened it and his father saw that he was quite alone with the telescope set up near the open window. 'I thought I heard people talking,' said his father. 'No you didn't.

Why don't you go away and leave me alone?' snapped David in reply.

It was a few weeks later, just after his eighteenth birthday, that David began to notice people staring at him. It happened mostly on the underground, but people at work sometimes looked at him strangely too. He knew that his colleagues were talking about him behind his back, so he decided to be very careful when he spoke to them. His inner hostility towards his colleagues became so strong at times that he found it hard to concentrate. He would often leave the office and shut himself in the toilet where he could call them names without them hearing. On one occasion a colleague walked into the toilets and heard David swearing to himself. News soon spread around the office that David was behaving oddly, and people began to avoid him.

One morning the supervisor called David into his office to point out that he was getting behind in his work. He had only just begun to offer some advice when David suddenly shouted at him, 'You're all the same here, talking about me and doing things to annoy me. They will get everyone in the end, you too. But they won't get me, I know about them!' David ran out of the supervisor's office and shut himself in the toilet.

A week later David was dismissed. The manager told him that the job was obviously not suitable for him, and that it was having a bad effect on his nerves. He advised him to find a job which did not demand so much concentration on figures.

On his way home from work that day David noticed people staring at him in the train. A few of the women coughed deliberately, and the men kept touching their noses. David felt a shiver run up and down his spine, and he began to tremble. Then he heard the sound. At first it was a soft whisper; the same unrecognisable voice he had heard before in his bedroom. 'Devil, Devil, I'm going to kill you! Dirty! Rotten! I can see you.' The voice grew louder and louder, repeating the same sentence over and over again, almost in tune with the sound of the wheels on the track. David looked up at the ventilation grill on the roof of the train. The voice came from that direction. Then he recognised it. It was his supervisor! So he was in it too. All the time he knew what was going on, and yet he said nothing. 'What should I do?'

thought David. 'Go back and kill him? No, there will be others. Look at them in the carriage. They are together in this. Look at that woman's eyes, they are fixed on me now. Look at her face, see how evil it is.'

The train pulled into the station and David jumped off quickly. He ran most of the way home; he would be safer there. When he arrived, his father was already in, and the table was set for the evening meal. 'Had a hard day son? You look worn out.' 'Poison!' David screamed, his eyes fixed on the plate of food his mother carried into the room. 'They'll poison you!' His mother was struck with horror as he snatched the plate from her and threw it at the wall. With a swipe of his hand he cleared several plates and glasses from the table, and ran upstairs shouting and screaming. His father chased after him.

In the ambulance, accompanied by his parents, David muttered to himself constantly. His mother, who was extremely upset, tried to speak to him, but his only reply was a meaningless jumble of words. 'We should have done something earlier,' she said to her husband as the vehicle stopped outside the admission ward. 'I knew he was behaving oddly, and I did tell you. This is terrible.'

David remained in hospital for three months. For the first two weeks he did nothing but sit in his side room muttering to his 'voices'. He would stare out of the window, sometimes grimacing and pointing to his visions. He refused to eat anything except potatoes. 'These are buried in the ground,' he said 'and could not be poisoned by the radiation.' During the acute phase of his illness David was always co-operative, and accepted his injections of chlorpromazine without protest. Towards the end of the third week his hallucinations became less frequent, and he was able to talk more rationally.

As David continued to improve, the doctor gradually reduced his large doses of chlorpromazine, and eventually prescribed fortnightly injections of Modecate. He soon became well enough to start working in the occupational therapy centre and to attend the regular ward meetings. Before he was discharged, the consultant saw his parents and impressed upon them the need for David to attend hospital regularly for his injections. David is now working as a clerk in a local shipping office. He keeps regular appointments with the doctor in the out-patients clinic, and calls into the ward for his injections.

CASE ILLUSTRATION 10: SCHIZOPHRENIA (iii)

Mabel Smith was the most outstanding patient in the ward. Every nurse got to know Mabel before any of the others. She wore the most elaborate, highly coloured clothes, and made it her business to introduce herself to every new nurse as soon a she arrived. 'My girl,' she would say, 'we hope you will show us more respect than the one who has left. We intend to see that she is dismissed!'

Mabel Smith believed that she was Queen Victoria. She wore a long dress made of bright blue silk, with frayed and discoloured lace trimmings at the collar and cuffs. Round her neck were several strings of imitation pearls which she refused to take off, even in the bath. Her hair was long, and during the day was held in a huge bun by numerous hair clips. On her head she wore a tiara made of plastic and decorated with imitation diamonds. This headpiece she had purchased in Woolworths for 1s 6d when on a ward outing to the seaside in 1967. The effect was completed by her brilliant red lipstick, so liberally used that it made her lips appear twice the normal size.

Unlike many patients with grandiose delusions, Mabel could make people feel that they were indeed inferior. She spoke to everyone in a superior tone that would have been comic had it not been so annoying. No one dared to laugh at Mabel. The merest hint of a smile, or a word which indicated disrespect, and Mabel would let out a stream of abuse. Her language would be so obscene that it never failed to produce results. When admonished for her language, which many times was pointed out to be inappropriate, she would say 'We do as we like. You are just a servant, remember that!'

Mabel would never answer to her real name. 'Your Majesty', 'Ma'am' or 'Queen Victoria' were the only titles to which she would respond. When signing her name to collect her weekly allowance, she would always write 'Victoria R.'. The ward sister would have to print 'Mabel Smith' after her signature when she had gone. If asked what happened to Mabel Smith, the reply was nearly always the same. 'She was killed when they discovered who I really was. I don't know much about her. She was a stupid girl, it had to be done.'

Mabel did very little work on the ward. She considered that most of the tasks were beneath her, although occasionally she would surprise everyone by setting the tables for the midday or evening meal. She refused to take part in industrial therapy, and would never go to the hospital socials or dances. In the evenings she would shut herself in her side room to sort through her belongings, which consisted largely of old newspapers, cigarette packets and toilet rolls. Her collection was jealously guarded, and no one could so much as touch anything without being met with abuse. She was totally involved in her private world, and any attempt to confront her with reality would arouse anger and hostility.

Like so many patients who have been in hospital for years, Mabel's early history is obscured by the passage of time. From her case notes, it is evident that she was first admitted in March 1932, suffering from what was called 'Delusional Insanity'. She had never married, although to this day she still refers to her husband 'Albert'. Until 1960 she was a Certified patient, but was given informal status as she was quite willing to remain in hospital. Early entries in her case notes state that she was hallucinated and destructive, and often had to be restrained. Today she is no longer physically aggressive, although she can sometimes be seen muttering to her 'voices'.

Mabel is currently taking 50 mg of Chlorpromazine three times a day, which she swallows without resentment. Recently she was interviewed by the doctor and a nursing officer with a view to placing her in a group home. It was decided not to take her out of the hospital setting, as her attitudes and grandiose behaviour would make communal living quite impossible for her.

QUESTIONS

1   Name two functional psychotic illnesses.

2 Give three symptoms of hypomania.
*3 Mention three features of depressive illness.
4 What treatments may be prescribed for a depressed patient?
5 Give three symptoms of schizophrenia.
6 How may the patient's personal hygiene be affected by schizophrenia?
7 How may industrial therapy help a schizophrenic patient?
8 What do you understand by the term 'stupor'?
9 How may a patient's emotions be affected by schizophrenia?
10 Give an example of a paranoid delusion.
11 What would you notice about a patient's behaviour that would lead you to believe he was hallucinated?
12 What treatments may be prescribed for schizophrenia?

* Reproduced by permission of The General Nursing Council for England and Wales.

Chapter 8

ORGANIC PSYCHOSES

The organic psychoses are a large group of serious mental illnesses caused by physical changes in the brain or body. The organic psychoses to be described here are senile dementia, the pre-senile dementias, arteriosclerotic dementia and the confusional states.

SENILE DEMENTIA

Dementia means irreversible loss of mental faculties. Senile dementia is a disease of old age in which mental faculties are seriously and irreversibly impaired.

Most of us will have been in close contact with old people at some time, and will be aware of their many peculiarities. Old folk like to re-tell stories of the distant past, but are often unable to remember the details of more recent events. They do not accept change easily, dislike new ideas and fashions, and find it difficult to learn new information. Emotional changes too are common in old age; old people do not share the enthusiasm of the younger generation (see Old Age, p 30). Senile dementia is an exaggeration of the natural features of old age. The illness produces marked changes in the patient's personality and behaviour.

Fortunately only a small percentage of old people suffer a serious loss of mental faculties. Senile dementia never occurs before the age of sixty-five years, and generally much later in life. The symptoms of the illness are caused by the death of large numbers of brain cells, particularly of the frontal lobes of the brain. The reason for the death of these cells in such large numbers is not known.

Signs and symptoms
Senile dementia usually begins slowly, but after only a few months

the patient may be seriously ill. The old person's relatives may first notice that something is wrong when he mislays possessions or becomes generally forgetful. Taps may be left running, doors and windows left open, and cigarettes may remain alight in ash trays or be allowed to drop on to the floor. The old person may forget to wash or shave, or find it hard to remember events that have only recently happened. At this stage of the illness the patient may try to conceal his **amnesia** by making up stories. Unable to remember where he has been during the morning, he may tell stories of long walks or of meeting friends. Making up excuses to conceal loss of memory is called **confabulation**.

As the illness continues, the change in the patient's personality and behaviour become more obvious. He may accuse people of stealing the articles he has mislaid, and become angry, irritable or tearful without good reason. He may not be able to recognise his surroundings, the time of day or even the date, and sometimes his own name will be forgotten. The failure to appreciate names, time and places is called **disorientation**.

The demented patient may become restless and confused, particularly at night. Often these confused, old people will potter aimlessly all night, sleeping only during the day; a condition known as **reversed sleep rhythm**.

Delusions, commonly of theft or ill treatment, and **auditory hallucinations** can make the demented patient very difficult to manage. At the same time his personal hygiene will deteriorate, and he may be unable to dress, wash or eat properly.

A decline in the patient's physical health accompanies his mental deterioration. Loss of weight, chest and urinary infections, and injuries due to falls are made worse by the patient's confusion. Incontinence and constipation occur, often because the patient is unable to find the lavatory. The picture of the patient in the final stage of the illness, physically ill, incontinent, aimlessly pottering and talking nonsense, is indeed sad. Patients suffering from senile dementia usually die from chest or other infections about two years after the onset of the disease.

Treatment
There is no effective treatment for senile dementia. Good nursing

care is essential to the patient's comfort and well-being. It is much better if the patient's relatives are able to look after him at home. Admission to hospital, with its strange surroundings, may only confuse him more. In many cases it may be possible to arrange for the patient to attend hospital for part of the day, allowing him to return home to familiar surroundings at night.

If the patient is admitted to hospital, the ward doctor will conduct a physical and mental examination. This is important, as the patient may be suffering from a physical disease or some other mental disorder. Frequently, elderly patients will require treatment for troublesome conditions such as chest and urinary infections, diabetes, heart disease or anaemia. Many doctors prescribe vitamins for elderly patients as a matter of course, as vitamin deficiency may be responsible for acute confusion (see p. 104. If the patient is restless, the doctor will generally prescribe a tranquillizer such as promazine, 50 mg three times daily. Insomnia is often best treated by giving the patient a warm drink, or even a tot of whisky before bed time. Old people react badly to hypnotic drugs, although they may sometimes be given if the patient is very restless. Barbiturate drugs, such as sodium amylobarbitone, should never be given to old people as they only increase confusion.

The patient's diet should contain adequate amounts of protein, fresh fruit, vegetables, milk and vitamins. A proper diet, which should not include many 'soft' foods, and regular exercise will help the patient's digestion and avoid constipation. Incontinent patients must be washed regularly if bedsores are to be prevented. Superficial cuts or bruises must receive prompt attention, and the necessary lotions and dressings must be applied immediately.

General management
In hospital it is important that the confused, elderly person is nursed in suitable accommodation. The ward should be small, well lit and easily ventilated. It should always be at ground level so that there is no risk of the elderly patient falling down stairs. Furniture and decorations should be chosen with care to make the ward as homely as possible. All clinical apparatus should be stored away except when it is in use.

Confused, elderly people are prone to falls, and care must be taken to reduce the risk of injury. Loose rugs and highly polished floors must never be allowed in a ward which houses old people. All floors should be covered with fitted carpets or 'non-slip' material. Furniture should be heavy or immobile, and wheel chairs must be secured if left in the vicinity of the patients.

Confused patients react badly to change, so a fixed daily routine is a necessary part of their nursing care. Unless the patient is physically ill he should not be allowed to remain in bed during the day. Apart from the risk of producing physical illness, confinement to bed will make the old person apathetic and even more confused. A daily programme should be drawn up, and this should include occupational activities and pastimes suitable for elderly people. All but the most seriously confused should be able to take part in at least some of the activities. A daily routine should not deprive the patient of his freedom. Likes and dislikes, personal habits and customs must be respected. If an elderly person enjoys reading in the afternoons rather than going for a walk, then he should be allowed to read.

The patient's friends and relations should be encouraged to visit as often as they can. Flexible visiting times always result in more visits for the patient, as relatives are not restricted to awkward visiting hours. A visit from a friend or relation, even if it is forgotten afterwards, can bring a great deal of joy to an old person confined to hospital. Quite often relations feel guilty about leaving the old person in the care of nurses. It will help the patient and his relatives if they can be encouraged to take him out for car rides or even home for short visits.

Attention to the patient's personal hygiene is of utmost importance. Whether he will require simple supervision or a lot of help from the nurse depends on his physical and mental condition. Regular washing and bathing should be encouraged. Oral hygiene is important, and the patient's eyes should be kept clean and free from mucus. Much can be done to make life more comfortable for the elderly patient by arranging for him to be supplied with dentures, spectacles and a hearing aid, if these are required.

Although senile dementia cannot be cured, the misery of the

disease can be greatly reduced by good nursing care. Skilled management of the patient is the most important, if not the only means of relieving this distressing condition of old age.

THE PRE-SENILE DEMENTIAS

The pre-senile dementias are a group of mental disorders which are very similar to senile dementia. They occur however before the age of sixty-five, often in the fifties or late forties. The illnesses are caused by the early death of large numbers of brain cells, and leave the patient mentally and physically feeble long before old age.

There are many types of pre-senile dementia, but all of them eventually leave the patients confused and physically ill. Quite often these patients suffer from epileptiform fits, paralyses and speech difficulties, in addition to the usual symptoms of dementia.

A type of pre-senile dementia called **Huntington's chorea** is worthy of special note. It is a hereditary disease passed from parent to child. The children of a person who suffers from Huntington's chorea stand a 50 per cent chance of developing the illness.

Huntington's chorea usually begins when the patient is between thirty and fifty years of age. It frequently commences with slight writhing and jerking movements of the face, shoulders or limbs, called **choreic movements**. These movements cannot be controlled by the patient. They become worse after a time and eventually involve almost the whole body, so that the patient walks only with difficulty, or is confined to bed.

The patient who suffers from Huntington's chorea may become seriously confused and disoriented, or he can remain quite aware of his surroundings with only slight amnesia. Often he will become bad tempered or even aggressive. In the early stage of the disease the patient may attempt suicide, particularly if he is aware of the true nature of his illness.

There is no successful medical treatment for any of the pre-senile dementias. No methods of preventing the illnesses are known. Children of known sufferers from Huntington's chorea are often informed by doctors of the risk to their offspring, and advised not to have children themselves.

The pre-senile dementias become worse over a period of time. The illnesses can last from two to fifteen years. Good nursing care is essential to the patient during this time, whether he is at home or in hospital. The general points on the management of confused patients (see p. 100) apply also to this group of mental disorders.

ARTERIOSCLEROTIC DEMENTIA

Arteriosclerotic dementia is a severe mental illness very similar to senile dementia (see p. 98). The symptoms of the illness are caused by the hardening and thickening of the arteries of the brain, **cerebral arteriosclerosis**. When this process occurs, the blood supply to the brain is reduced, and brain cells die in large numbers. Arteriosclerotic dementia is usually a disease of old age.

It is often very difficult to distinguish between arteriosclerotic dementia and senile dementia. Arteriosclerotic dementia develops more slowly. The patient may be very confused at some times, and at others only slightly forgetful. At the beginning of the illness the patient may know that he is losing his memory, and will try to conceal this by using note books and diaries. A few patients suffer from epileptiform fits or paralyses. In the late stages of the disease the patient will be confused, disoriented and physically weak.

There is no successful treatment for arteriosclerotic dementia. The points on the general management of patients suffering from senile dementia also apply to this illness.

ACUTE CONFUSIONAL STATES

Acute confusion, when the patient is disoriented and often mentally excited, is sometimes called **delirium**. There are many causes of this condition but the most usual are:

1 Infections which cause the patient's temperature to rise, e.g. pneumonia, influenza, septicaemia.

2   Diseases of, or injury to the brain, e.g. cerebral tumour, meningitis, head injury, cerebral haemorrhage.
3   The poisonous effects of drugs and gases, especially barbiturates, amphetamines, alcohol and carbon monoxide.
4   The toxic (poisonous) effects of renal and liver failure.
5   A reduction of the blood supply, and therefore oxygen, to the brain (**cerebral anoxia**), commonly due to heart and respiratory disease and haemorrhage.
6   Vitamin deficiency, especially vitamin B_{12}.

Signs and symptoms
In acute confusion the patient's level of consciousness is disturbed. This is called **clouding of consciousness**. The patient will not know where he is, and will find it difficult to understand what is happening around him. He may become easily upset by people and objects which he cannot recognise. Delirious patients are often visually hallucinated, and illusions are extremely common.

It may be very difficult to understand what an acutely confused patient is saying, for his talk is sometimes rambling and incoherent. He lives in a frightening world, full of strange happenings and unrecognisable objects. Because of this he will be afraid, suspicious or even terrified.

Treatment
Most acutely confused patients recover completely once the cause of the illness has been treated. A thorough physical examination by the doctor will be necessary to establish the cause. The appropriate treatment for the physical illness must begin as soon as possible.

While the physical illness is being treated, a great deal can be done to improve the patient's mental condition. Delirious patients can become exhausted and die, so adequate nourishment and sleep are important aspects of treatment. The patient should be gently persuaded to take small meals and frequent drinks of milk, water or squash. The amount of fluid the patient drinks must be accurately recorded. This is particularly important when his temperature is raised. If he is very confused it may be convenient to give him drinks of liquid food such as Complan in place of the small meals.

The patient should be encouraged to rest as much as possible. He will be less confused if he is kept away from noise and activity. It is often better if the patient can be nursed in a side room, but this should always be evenly lit, even at night. Shadows and darkness only increase the fear of the confused patient. A nurse should always remain with him, and must be ready to reassure him in a kindly, soothing voice. It should always be remembered that the way in which the nurse deals with all confused patients has the greatest effect upon their behaviour and well-being.

CHRONIC CONFUSIONAL STATES

A chronic confusional state may follow acute confusion. This can happen when the treatment of the physical illness has not been successful, or when the brain has been damaged by disease. The serious complications of infections such as meningitis and syphilis have been largely overcome by the antibiotic drugs, and brain damage as a result of these infections is now rare. In the case of syphilis it only occurs when the patient has not been treated. Chronic confusional states are now most commonly caused by brain damage as a result of accident, strokes, cerebral tumours and poisoning with drugs, especially alcohol.

Signs and symptoms
The degree of confusion varies widely. Some patients are only mildly confused, while others are severely demented. All confused patients suffer from memory impairment, and many make up convincing stories to conceal their forgetfulness. Very often the patient is subject to outbursts of anger or tearfulness, and may find difficulty in controlling his feelings. For this reason, confused patients should always be treated with the utmost tact and gentleness. A decline in personal hygiene is quite common, although some patients maintain a high degree of cleanliness while not fully realising where they are or the time of day. In addition to the mental symptoms, and depending on the cause of

the illness, the patient may suffer from physical disabilities such as paralysis, speech defects, epileptic fits and heart disease.

Treatment

It is quite wrong to assume that the outlook is hopeless for all chronically confused patients. Depending on the cause and extent of the disease, an active rehabilitation programme can help some patients to lead useful lives outside hospital. The success of re-training programmes for patients with brain damage as a result of strokes or head injury have proved this beyond doubt. However, for the seriously demented patient, the most that can usually be done is to make his life as comfortable as possible by providing good nursing care (see the management of confused patients, p. 100).

CASE ILLUSTRATION 11: SENILE DEMENTIA

'We really must get the doctor to see your mother', said Mr Johnson to his wife. 'She really is getting worse, you know, and you are looking so tired these days. If something isn't done soon you'll be ill yourself. You can't go on like this.' Mrs Johnson had just explained to her husband how she had arrived home from the shops that morning to find the whole house smelling of gas. When she had asked her mother what had happened, all she said was, 'I don't know, but there's a funny smell in here.' She had turned the gas cooker on, forgotten to light it, and then had forgotten that the gas was escaping. 'I know what the doctor will say,' replied Mrs Johnson. 'He will want to send mother to that hospital outside town, and you know how she hates hospitals.' 'Maybe he won't,' said Mr Johnson. 'Possibly there is some other way of helping her. In any case you don't have to send her anywhere, but it would be a good idea to ask the doctor for advice. I'll telephone him from work tomorrow morning.'

Mrs Greene had celebrated her eightieth birthday a few weeks ago. It is true that she had been forgetting little things for some time, but that was not unusual for someone of her age. She was no problem at home, and she would always set the tables and prepare the food for her daughter to cook when she returned from work.

The three people lived quite happily together; there were none of the tensions so often found in a house where an elderly relative is cared for.

Three months ago the situation began to change. Mrs Greene suddenly stopped setting the table and preparing the food for the evening meal. 'Where have you been?' she would ask her daughter when she came home from work. Mrs Greene was losing her memory rapidly. She began to leave taps running during the day, and one evening Mrs Johnson arrived home to find the kitchen completely flooded. Her mother was upstairs sorting clothes in her wardrobe.

After a few weeks Mrs Johnson decided to give up work to look after her mother. It was obvious that she was not eating during the day, and besides it was no longer safe to leave her alone all day. At first Mrs Green did not need a great deal of looking after. Her daughter stayed at home only to ensure that she did not do anything silly, and to prepare her a midday meal. After only two weeks she became more dependent, following her daughter from room to room, and insisting that she should listen to the same stories repeated over and over again. Whenever she went out Mrs Johnson would return to find her mother crying, and wandering about aimlessly.

Mr Johnson telephoned the doctor as he had promised his wife, and he called to see Mrs Greene the same evening. He told Mrs Johnson that he was going to ask a psychiatrist to visit her mother, and a week later a consultant from the local psychiatric hospital arrived. He asked Mrs Greene a lot of questions, mainly to test her memory and orientation. The psychiatrist was convinced that Mrs Greene was quite seriously demented, but wanted his diagnosis confirmed. He could see that Mrs Johnson was not prepared to let her mother go into hospital, and so he suggested that she should spend each week day in the psychiatric day hospital, returning home each evening. This would provide some relief for Mrs Johnson, and allow him to carry out the necessary investigations. Mrs Johnson willingly agreed to this, relieved that her mother could still come home at night.

On the first morning Mrs Johnson accompanied her mother in the ambulance to the day hospital. It seemed a pleasant enough building, specially designed for elderly people. It was cheerfully decorated, the other patients were friendly and not at all as she had feared. When she arrived, some of the nurses were giving the patients cups of tea, and helpers were setting up some tables for a handiwork session. Mrs Johnson quickly saw that her mother would be happy here. There were other people to talk to, nurses to take care of her and see that she came to no harm, and interesting ways of passing the time. Her belief was confirmed by the sister, who explained the various activities in the unit and what her mother would be doing that day. 'You have no need to worry, Mrs Johnson,' said the sister. 'Your mother will be well taken care of.'

It was three weeks later, when Mrs Greene had settled into the routine of going to the hospital each day, that the consultant sent for her daughter. 'I think your mother has settled in well, Mrs Johnson,' said the consultant. 'She appears to be quite happy here during the day.' 'Yes indeed, doctor,' replied Mrs Johnson, 'and she is virtually no trouble at home now. I think that coming here during the day helps to keep her mind occupied.' 'I'm afraid that the news isn't all good though, Mrs Johnson,' the consultant continued. 'The tests we have done show that your mother isn't likely to get much better. There will come a time – and I can't say how soon this will be – when she will need more care than she does now.' 'What do you mean exactly?' asked Mrs Johnson. 'Well, she has a mental illness which is progressive. By that I mean she is likely to get worse. At the moment she can remember many things, mainly from the past. As I'm sure you know, she is unable to remember recent events, such as what she was doing yesterday or what she had to eat this morning. As it is now she can recognise her surroundings, even though she cannot remember their names. I'm afraid there is a likelihood that her memory will get worse, and that she will become more and more confused. If this happens, you are going to find it very difficult to care for her at home, even in the evenings and at week-ends. She will then need expert care and attention which can only be given in hospital.' 'You mean that she will need to be admitted to hospital as an in-patient?' asked Mrs Johnson. 'Yes, I'm afraid so. But until that happens she can continue to come here each day. It will really be up to you to decide Mrs Johnson. You must ask to see me if things become too difficult for you at home.' Mrs Johnson left the hospital feeling disappointed, even though the doctor had only confirmed what she had feared all along. Perhaps, when the time came, her mother would not mind staying in a place she knew, which, after all, could provide the expert care that she was unable to give at home.

CASE ILLUSTRATION 12: ACUTE CONFUSIONAL STATE

'It's Mr Conway, Sister, he wants to find his wife,' said the nurse as she passed the sister's office, the patient's arm linked to hers. He was dressed in pyjamas, the coat of which he had somehow managed to put on back to front. The nurse walked with Mr Conway through the ward and helped him to sit on his bed. It was difficult to get his pyjama coat off and replace it correctly. The patient tried to co-operate, but kept waving his arms in a way which only led to entanglement. After some time the nurse succeeded and got Mr Conway into bed. He put his head on the pillow and said straight away, 'I think it's time to get up.' 'No, Mr Conway, I want you to stay in bed,' said the nurse. 'The doctor says you are to stay in bed and not go wandering around like this.' 'Doctor? I don't like doctors. Where is my wife? Who do you think you are? Get away from me!' The nurse left Mr Conway quickly. Only yesterday she had seen him throw a bottle at a nurse, narrowly missing her head.

The nurse returned to the office where the sister was already speaking to the doctor on the telephone. 'Will you come to see Mr Conway, please? He is very restless again, and probably needs sedation.' Replacing the receiver, she said to the nurse, 'Go and fetch Nurse Smith and try to keep Mr Conway in bed until the doctor arrives.' She removed the patient's case folder from the cabinet and placed them on her desk.

Mr Conway had been admitted to hospital five days ago, after falling from a ladder while decorating his house. He had suffered an injury to his head, and remained deeply unconscious for forty-eight hours. He recovered slowly, but became very confused, talking incoherently. Noise and people passing his bed seemed to disturb him, and he tried to attack the nursing staff on several occasions. He was placed in a side room where noise and movement would not upset him so easily. Yesterday he recovered sufficiently to be able to get out of bed, but he was still very confused and restless.

The doctor arrived just in time to see Mr Conway struggling with the nurses to get out of bed. 'I want to see my wife,' he said angrily. 'Your wife will be coming soon,' replied the doctor. 'No, she won't. She doesn't know where I am. Who are you anyway?' The doctor prescribed an injection of chlorpromazine for Mr Conway, and with the sister's tact and persuasion it was given without too much fuss. Soon after the injection he calmed down and eventually went off to sleep.

During the days that followed Mr Conway improved rapidly. He became less restless and confused, and eventually realised that he was in hospital. An electro-encephalograph confirmed that he had suffered no permanent brain damage, and he was discharged three weeks later, fully recovered. He remembers nothing of the events which led up to his injury, and can only remember the latter part of his stay in hospital.

QUESTIONS

1 What do you understand by the term 'organic psychosis'?
2 What is the meaning of the word 'dementia'?
3 Name three types of dementia.
4 Give four symptoms of senile dementia.
5 What do you understand by the term 'disorientation'?
6 What changes take place in the sleep pattern of patients suffering from senile dementia?
7 What types of delusion are commonly found in senile dementia?
8 Name three physical conditions from which demented patients commonly suffer.
9 State four measures that can be taken to reduce the risk of injuries in a ward for elderly patients.
10 What measures can be taken to reduce the fear and confusion of a delirious patient?

Chapter 9

PSYCHOPATHIC DISORDER

The term **psychopathic disorder** is used to describe a group of conditions which are not regarded as neurotic or psychotic. They are abnormalities of character and personality rather than well-defined mental illnesses.

A **psychopath** is a person who continually behaves in an irresponsible or aggressive way, without regard to the effect his behaviour has upon other people. He does not learn by his mistakes, and punishment will not deter him. He is sent to hospital when it is felt that medical treatment may have some effect on his behaviour.

A psychopath can be of high or average intelligence, or mentally subnormal. Quite often he will have experienced a disturbed, unhappy childhood. His abnormal behaviour first becomes obvious in adolescence or even in late childhood.

The most outstanding feature of a psychopath's character is his **antisocial behaviour**. He will not like work, and in order to live, may borrow or steal money or sponge on relatives. The rules of society, by which most of us abide, are ignored by the psychopath. He resents control, and reacts with hostility to authority and discipline. He has no consideration for other people unless courtesy and respect will work to his advantage.

A psychopath likes to impress other people. He may tell stories of daring pursuits, or financial achievements, none of which contain the slightest grain of truth. This shameless story-telling is called **pathological lying**. Quite often a psychopath will appear charming, well-dressed and confident. He may take an apparently genuine interest in other people, and succeed in gaining their trust. Having done so he will proceed to use them to his own advantage, and of course abandon them once his purpose is served.

A psychopath will try to get what he wants immediately,

without considering the views and feelings of others. If he cannot get his own way he is likely to become angry or violent. In an argument he is always in the right, and even violence will be justified in his eyes.

Psychopaths are weak-willed individuals who dislike more mature, stable people. If they marry, their partner is usually just as irresponsible. Their associates are of a similar character, and the saying 'birds of a feather flock together' is, in the case of psychopaths, perfectly true.

Psychopathic people sometimes conflict with the law. They may be sent to prison for such crimes as stealing, drug peddling, blackmail or violent assault. Prison sentences do nothing to correct their behaviour, and they are often sent to hospital when all else has failed.

There are three types of psychopathic disorder. They are referred to as:

The **aggressive** type, who is usually of low intelligence. He can become aggressive and violent without the slightest reason.

The **hysterical** type, who behaves in a theatrical way. He loves to draw attention to himself, and displays intense, insincere emotions.

The **inadequate** type, who is irresponsible and weak-willed. He is unable to cope with life's problems, and demands help and support from others.

Treatment

Most doctors agree that a psychopathic disorder is extremely difficult to treat. The patient will improve only when he has learned a more acceptable way of behaving. Treatment is designed to teach him new patterns of behaviour.

There are two methods of treatment. One involves firm discipline, when the patient must abide by definite rules. When he behaves reasonably he is rewarded, and when he breaks the rules he is punished in some way. This method of treatment is most effective when the patient is legally detained in hospital and cannot discharge himself. The other method of treatment encourages the patient to see his own mistakes and deal with the consequences of his behaviour. It is usually carried out in special units for psychopaths, with patients and staff making the rules together. Group therapy and discussions help the patient to deal with problems in a more adult and mature way.

Both methods of treatment claim some success, but the fact is most psychopaths remain irresponsible or aggressive in spite of treatment. However, many become less aggressive towards middle age. If they can avoid serious trouble with the law, they can eventually become acceptable if not responsible, citizens.

General management

The psychopathic patient can present many problems in hospital. Psychopaths are past masters at stirring up feelings of resentment and jealousy. They will use every weakness they can find in staff relationships to destroy trust and good will. Because of this the nurse must never discuss other members of staff or patients with a psychopath, no matter how genuine and interested he may seem. He will only use personal information to destroy relationships and create ill feeling.

A psychopath may try to use the relationship he has made with a nurse to his advantage. He will often attempt to persuade, blackmail or threaten a nurse into doing what he asks or letting him have his own way. It is not uncommon for this to happen just when the nurse is beginning to feel that at last she is able to help him. Whenever a psychopath uses these tactics to get his own way, the nurse must discuss the problem with the ward team or someone in authority. This problem will not arise so easily if she tells other members of staff of her relationship with the patient, and does not attempt to deal with him alone.

A psychopath will try to persuade or bully other patients into doing what he wants. Often he will succeed in getting them to take the blame for his misdeeds. Weak and easily-led patients should be encouraged to form relationships with other, more stable people. This can be a difficult task, as a psychopath can present a likeable personality and attract a great deal of 'hero worship'.

When a psychopath attacks another person it is generally someone smaller or weaker than himself. He may become violent for no apparent reason, or simply because he cannot get his own way. (The problem of violence is discussed in Chapter 14.) Violent, psychopathic patients should not be nursed in a ward in which there are elderly or infirm people.

Whatever form of treatment a psychopathic patient is receiving, he will generally behave more responsibly towards calm, friendly people. The nurse should never adopt an authoritarian or aggressive attitude, even when the patient's hostility is directed at her. If the psychopath knows that the nurse cannot be black-mailed or manipulated, but is still prepared to help him, then his relationship with her can be of some value. Only through reasonably stable relationships can a psychopath learn to behave in a more responsible and acceptable way.

CASE ILLUSTRATION 13: PSYCHOPATHIC DISORDER

Roger sat in the armchair and lit himself a cigarette. He inhaled deeply and blew a cloud of smoke across the doctor's desk. 'I suppose you're going to tell that I've got to go,' he announced, staring at the ceiling. 'No,' replied the doctor, 'I am not.' 'Pity,' said Roger, 'I hate it here with all these crazy people. Even the nurses are cracked! I don't know what good being here is doing me.' 'You are here on a Probation Order Roger, and if you leave the probation officer will want to know why.' 'Yes, there's that to it, I guess,' said Roger, taking another long draw of his cigarette. 'It's a question of here or jail isn't it? At least I can go out here to get away from the head cases.' 'I think you are right when you say that being here isn't helping you,' said the doctor. 'I am going to send you to another ward which I am sure will be better for you.' Roger sat upright, and for the first time fixed his eyes on the doctor. 'What ward? I'm not going to another ward!'

Roger Jacobs had been sent to hospital under a Probation Order six weeks previously, after appearing in court on a charge of possessing cannabis. This was his latest offence in almost ten years of criminal activities, dating back to just after his fifteenth birthday. His first offence was taking and driving away a motor vehicle, and for this he was fined. Only three months later he appeared in court again, charged with a similar offence, and was put on probation for a year. Between then and his seventeenth birthday he had no fewer than six offences involving motor vehicles, and at last the magistrate sent him to a detention centre for six months. At the centre he was always getting involved in fights and causing arguments among the other boys, so much that the head master recorded that he was 'by far the most disruptive influence in the centre'.

After leaving the centre he found himself a job on a building site, but was dismissed after only three weeks over, as he puts it 'some stupid argument with the foreman'. In fact, the foreman told him to 'pull his weight' and an argument ensued. Roger punched him in the face and, knocking him to the ground, set about kicking his head. The foreman spent several days in hospital recovering from his injuries. This 'argument' resulted in what was to be the first of several court appearances on assault charges. Roger had a succession of jobs over a four-year period, none of which he could hold for more than a few months. He either left because he didn't like them or was fired for arguing or stealing.

Until last year Roger lived at home with his parents. He was always at loggerheads with his father, and on more than one occasion came to blows with him. Roger maintained that he 'would never hit his old man', but the facts do not accord with his statement. During his periods of unemployment he would ask his mother for money, and she was too afraid of her son to refuse. It was after an argument with his father over borrowing money to buy drink that Roger left home. He went to live with a friend, a woman who was almost twice his age. As Roger says, 'she was good for a few bob'. While living with her he supplemented his income by selling cannabis and heroin in pubs and on the streets. He had no intention of ever working again. 'Why should I work?' he would say. 'I can get almost as much on the dole, and in other ways. Only mugs go to work.'

Roger had been a problem ever since he first arrived in hospital. Although he was never physically aggressive to the nursing staff, he would go out of his way to get involved in fights with other patients. If he was not fighting himself, he certainly had something to do with any disturbance in the ward. He insisted on leaving and returning to the hospital at all hours of the day and night, and often came back drunk. He avoided doing his share of the work by enlisting the sympathy of the other patients, or if that failed, threatening them. The doctor was quite right. Little could be done to help him in that ward.

'Look, Roger,' continued the doctor, 'I am going to send you to a ward where you will have more freedom than you have here. But you will have more responsibility too. You will find the other patients have a good deal to say in the running of the ward, and you will be expected to contribute.' Roger agreed to go when he was assured that he was not being sent to a long-stay ward in the main part of the hospital. In fact, his new ward was run along the lines of a therapeutic community, with the patients taking most of the decisions and setting most of the rules.

Roger Jacobs remained in his new ward for three months. Records show that after initial difficulty he settled down, and was far more co-operative than he had been previously. He announced one day at the group meeting that he was going to find himself a job. That afternoon he went out to look for employment, and did not return. His probation officer was informed, but Roger has never been seen or heard of since.

QUESTIONS

1 What do you understand by the term 'psychopathic disorder'?
2 Name the three types of psychopathic disorder.
3 State three ways in which a psychopathic patient can be a problem in a psychiatric hospital ward.
4 Mention one way in which a psychopathic patient may react to authority or frustration.
5 What should the nurse do if she is becoming too involved with a psychopathic patient?
6 State one form of treatment for psychopathic patients.

Chapter 10

DRUG DEPENDENCE

It is not unusual to find in every psychiatric hospital a few patients who are seeking help to give up taking drugs. These patients are not always mentally ill, but they may benefit from the special care a psychiatric hospital can give. For this reason the nurse should know of the problem of drug dependence and the various treatments available for it.

Drugs of various kinds have been used by man for thousands of years. They have been taken to relieve pain, cure illnesses or simply for pleasure. Today, most drugs are used only for medical reasons, although a few are taken for the pleasure they bring the user.

Tea, coffee, tobacco and alcohol are drugs commonly taken for pleasure. They can be purchased freely, and of course their use is not against the law. Tea and coffee, which contain the drug caffeine, are used by many people as a stimulant. Tobacco, which contains the drug nicotine, is said to have a soothing effect upon those who smoke it. Alcohol, in the form of wine, beer and spirit, is used to relieve tension, help conversation and produce a feeling of well-being.

Most other drugs are manufactured only for medical use. Many of these are available only on prescription from a doctor. A few people misuse some of these restricted drugs by taking them for pleasure rather than for their intended purpose. The restricted drugs most frequently misused are barbiturates, amphetamines, morphine, heroin, cocaine and the drugs which produce hallucinations such as lysergic acid diethylamide (L.S.D.).

Some drugs are considered to be **habit forming**, and others **addictive**. A habit forming drug is one which we take because we like it and may become accustomed to using. Tea, coffee and tobacco are examples of habit forming drugs. An addictive drug is one which the user comes to depend on physically and emotionally. The drug cannot be given up without physical and psychological discomfort.

A drug addict is a person who takes drugs to excess, or for a purpose for which they were not intended. He has an **intense craving** for the effects of the drug he uses. As time passes he needs to take more and more of the drug to experience the same effects. This need for greater amounts of the drug is called **tolerance**. When he stops taking the drug he experiences various mental and physical effects which are often very unpleasant. These feelings of discomfort are called **withdrawal symptoms**. A person is not truly addicted to a drug unless he experiences intense craving, tolerance and withdrawal symptoms.

It has been suggested that people who become addicted to drugs have a special type of personality, or even that they are mentally ill or psychopathic. It is true that some mentally ill or psychopathic people become addicted to drugs, but most addicts cannot be diagnosed in this way. The only feature drug addicts seem to have in common is their wish to avoid facing up to the real world.

Many people who misuse drugs first do so in adolescence. The drugs they take may help to ease the problems of growing up and the difficulties of adjusting to adult behaviour. Of course, in the long run drugs only increase these difficulties and make matters worse. Adolescents need to express themselves as individuals and may do so by becoming hostile towards parents and others in authority. Taking drugs is a way of rebelling against authority. Some people begin to misuse drugs later in life, often as a relief from tension, depression or boredom. Thousands of middle-aged women are dependent on barbiturate drugs in the United Kingdom, and addiction to alcohol is common in middle age.

Young people who take drugs regularly often mix only with other drug-takers. Large groups of drug users can influence other young people, and this often happens in schools, colleges and universities. Addicts become friendly with each other because of the support this gives them, and also because they can buy and sell drugs more easily this way. Serious drug-takers use their own terms to describe the 'drug scene'. A list of the more popular words used by addicts, and their meanings, is given on pp. 124–5.

Many people who take drugs are able to work, and lead reasonably normal lives. Others become addicted, lose their jobs and turn to crime in order to pay for the drugs. Some, particularly those who take a mixture of drugs, and those who are homeless, become physically ill and may die.

The drugs which are frequently misused are often referred to as 'soft' and 'hard'. 'Hard' drugs are addictive or extremely habit forming, while the 'soft' drugs are habit forming and may be addictive. The problem of addiction to alcohol is discussed separately (see p. 125).

AMPHETAMINES

Amphetamines, more commonly known as 'pep pills', are stimulant drugs. They give the user extra energy and a feeling of well-being. At one time they were used as antidepressants or to curb the appetite of overweight people. Amphetamines are now seldom prescribed for medical use, and their supply is restricted under Schedule 2 of the Misuse of Drugs Regulations, 1973.

The brand names of the amphetamine group of drugs are Benzedrine, Dexedrine, Durophet and Methedrine. They are all habit forming drugs. People who misuse them do not become truly addicted, but find great difficulty in giving them up. Amphetamines are often used by people who want to stay awake for long periods or by those who regularly go to all-night parties.

A person who takes large amounts of amphetamine over a period will suffer from restlessness, insomnia and loss of weight. He may also become irritable and paranoid, and in some cases develop a schizophrenic-like illness known as 'amphetamine psychosis'. When he stops taking the drug, he will experience a 'come down', which is really severe depression.

BARBITURATES

Until recently, barbiturates were the most popular of the 'sleeping pills'. They have been used since the beginning of this century, but only for the past fifteen years have they been misused by young people.

Young people who take barbiturate drugs like to stay awake and 'enjoy' the effects of them. They sedate the user and give him a feeling of drunkenness. Indeed, the effects of barbiturates are very similar to the effects of alcohol. Many people who are addicted to other drugs also take barbiturates. Often they are taken by injection under non-sterile conditions, for example, by mixing crushed tablets with tap water.

The misuse of barbiturates by middle-aged people is widespread in the United Kingdom. However, these people do not take the drugs to remain awake, but take excess amounts of them in order to sleep. Many find it quite impossible to sleep without the aid of barbiturates.

The barbiturate drugs are addictive, although they are not regarded by addicts as 'hard' drugs. Many doctors will no longer prescribe barbiturates for insomnia, but prefer to give the patient one of the 'non-barbiturate' sleeping tablets (see p. 181).

CANNABIS

Cannabis, or Indian Hemp has been used in various parts of the world for thousands of years. It is not used as a medicine in the United Kingdom, and its supply is restricted under Schedule 4 of the Misuse of Drugs Regulations, 1973.

The common names for cannabis are hash, pot, weed and marijuana. Those who take the drug always smoke it in the form of a cigarette, called a 'joint' or 'reefer'. Its users hold that it is more pleasant and less dangerous than alcohol. The effect cannabis has upon the user varies. Some people say that it helps them to appreciate the 'true' meanings of pictures and music. Others say that objects look more beautiful and conversation has more meaning under its influence.

Large quantities of cannabis can cause drowsiness and mild confusion. Apart from stimulating appetite, moderate use of the drug seems to produce no ill effects. It is not a drug of addiction, and is probably no more habit forming than tobacco. Even so, possession of cannabis is illegal in the United Kingdom and other Western countries. Although it is against the law there is little doubt that the drug is widely used. In many parts of the United

States, and in Canada changes in the law are being considered to reduce the penalties for possessing cannabis. In the United Kingdom arguments for and against a change in the law can be read in newspapers from time to time.

THE OPIATES

The drug opium is produced from the opium poppy which is grown in the hotter regions of the world. Opium has been used for thousands of years for both pleasure and relief from pain. The drugs derived from opium such as morphine, heroin and codeine, and other synthetic drugs are used widely as major analgesics today. They are restricted under Schedule 2 of the Misuse of Drugs Regulations, 1973.

Taken for pleasure, the opiates give the user a feeling of euphoria and extreme well-being. Generally, they are taken by intravenous injection, although sometimes orally. These drugs are extremely addictive. A user can become dependent on them after only a few days, needing larger and larger doses as time goes by. He will then become entirely preoccupied with the drug and lose interest in work, food and personal hygeine.

COCAINE

Cocaine is produced from the coca shrub of South America. It is used medically as a local anaesthetic, and its supply is restricted under Schedule 2 of the Misuse of Drugs Regulations, 1973.

People who misuse the drug take it in the form of a powder which they sniff. Used in this way cocaine is a powerful stimulant, and gives extra energy. It is not a drug of addiction, but can be extremely habit forming. Cocaine is often used by people addicted to the opiates.

THE HALLUCINOGENS

A hallucinogen is a drug which produces hallucinations. The two most common hallucinogens are mescaline and lysergic acid diethylamide (L.S.D.). Both drugs have been used medically to treat the mentally ill, but only under very special conditions. The hallucinogens are restricted under Schedule 4 of the Misuse of Drugs Regulations, 1973.

Mescaline and L.S.D. are commonly known as 'psychedelic' drugs. The word psychedelic means mind-opening, and describes the peculiar effects of the drugs. People who misuse them do so to 'see into their minds', or to experience the strange happenings and thoughts the drugs produce. Such an experience under the influence of mescaline or L.S.D. is called a 'trip'.

The hallucinogens are not drugs of addiction, although some people get used to taking them. They are used mostly by the more educated young people, and in colleges and universities. The drugs can be dangerous as they take the user away from reality. There have been reports of some young people falling under trains or jumping from windows under the effects of the hallucinogens.

Withdrawal symptoms

The physical and psychological discomforts a user feels when he stops taking his drug are called withdrawal symptoms. With some drugs the symptoms are quite mild, but with others they are very distressing and dangerous.

People who suddenly stop taking the habit forming drugs such as tobacco, cannabis and amphetamine do not experience physical withdrawal symptoms. After some time without the drug they may become depressed or irritable, but these symptoms quickly disappear. Habit forming drugs can be given up suddenly without ill effect, but the user must want to give them up.

The barbiturate group of drugs produce serious withdrawal symptoms. After about ten hours without the drug, the addict may complain of severe headache. Later he will begin to tremble and his muscles will twitch uncontrollably. Epileptiform fits commonly occur, and some addicts become delirious if deprived of the drug for many hours. If a patient is known to be addicted to barbiturates he should be observed closely. If any of the above symptoms appear the doctor must be informed at once as the risk of death from barbiturate withdrawal is high.

People who are addicted to the opiate group of drugs also experience withdrawal symptoms. These are not as dangerous as barbiturate withdrawal symptoms, but are extremely unpleasant. After about twelve hours without the drug the addict becomes sleepy, perspires heavily and yawns almost constantly. Later he becomes wide awake and develops cramplike pains in his back and limbs. He will complain of feeling extremely cold, and may ask for blankets. These symptoms continue for about three days. Although they are extremely unpleasant, the symptoms do not persuade the addict to give up the drug for good.

Treatment
Treatment involves getting the patient to give up his drugs, and once he has given them up, to help him live without them. With modern care and treatment, weaning the patient from the drug is not difficult. The difficulty is in getting the patient to see the need for treatment, and afterwards, keeping him from using the drug again. This difficulty applies to the users of all drugs, from the least habit forming to the most addictive.

People who use the habit forming drugs, once they want to give them up, can do so suddenly. They will, however, need a great deal of support and encouragement from those who look after them. The doctor may prescribe antidepressant drugs to those people who have stopped taking amphetamines, to see them over the short period of depression.

Those who are addicted to the barbiturate and opiate drugs are best treated in hospital or a special treatment centre. Barbiturate addicts cannot be suddenly deprived of their drug, and the dose must be gradually reduced over a period of weeks. Patients who are receiving treatment for barbiturate addiction must be closely observed to ensure that they are not obtaining extra supplies. The treatment is designed to wean the patient from the drug, ensuring that he does not experience withdrawal symptoms.

Treatment for addiction to the opiate drugs is best carried out in special drug treatment centres. Here the patient can receive treatment on a daily basis while remaining at work or living at home. The patient is first of all assessed by the doctor so that he can prescribe a minimum dose which keeps him free from withdrawal symptoms. Weaning the patient from his drug is carried out over a period, and the dosage is reduced slowly. Often the patient is given the drug methadone to replace his usual drug. This is because it is easier to reduce the amount of methadone without ill effects.

The outlook for drug addicts is fairly good if they can find a job which interests them, and have good relationships with people who do not abuse drugs. Unfortunately many drug addicts are unemployed, homeless and associate only with other addicts. Their circumstances make it very difficult for them to live without taking drugs for very long. However, a number of addicts decide to give up drugs themselves when they reach their late twenties or early thirties. Perhaps this is because at last they see the foolishness of their actions which can lead only to chronic illness and early death.

A LIST OF WORDS USED BY DRUG ADDICTS

Acid	= L.S.D.
Bennies	= benzedrine
Black bomber	= durophet
Burn	= smoke
Buzz	= stimulating effect of drugs
C	= cocaine
Coke	= cocaine
Cold turkey	= sudden withdrawal from addictive drugs
Come down	= wearing off of the effects of drugs
Dex	= dexedrine
Dry out	= withdraw from drugs slowly
Goof balls	= barbiturate drugs
Grass	= cannabis
H	= heroin
Hash	= cannabis
High	= under the influence of drugs
Joint	= a cigarette containing cannabis
Main line	= inject a drug intravenously

Meth	= methedrine
Pot	= cannabis
Push	= to sell drugs
Score	= to obtain drugs
Shot	= injection
Sleepers	= barbiturate drugs
Stoned	= under the influence of cannabis
Stuff	= drugs
Trip	= an experience with L.S.D.
Weed	= cannabis

ALCOHOLISM

Alcoholism is addiction to the drug alcohol. It is the most common form of addiction in the Western world, and the number of alcoholics is increasing year by year. Although alcohol is freely available, addiction to it is no less serious than addiction to the 'hard' drugs such as heroin and morphine.

Most people who drink alcohol for pleasure restrict their intake. Occasional drinks with meals, in the evenings or to celebrate special events are in most cases harmless. The average person finds no difficulty in going without alcohol, and only rarely drinks to excess. The alcoholic regularly drinks far too much. He is quite unable to continue for many hours without drink, even if it means drinking alone or at an unacceptable time of day. The alcoholic does not drink simply because he is weak willed. He is physically dependent upon alcohol in the same way as the drug addict is dependent upon his supply of heroin.

Most alcoholics start to drink heavily at a fairly early age. They may be addicted to alcohol for years before they finally accept treatment. Even then they seek help generally because of physical illness, family or financial problems, rather than from a desire to give up drink.

Alcoholism has serious consequences both for the drinker and his family. An alcoholic is seldom sober as he needs to drink large amounts throughout the day. He will need a drink early in the morning before going to work, and quite possibly a drink when he gets there. Lunch time is spent in a bar, and food is far less important than drink. Even small problems at work cannot be dealt with without 'a quick drink' beforehand. In the evenings, whether he is out or at home, drinking is the main, if not the only entertainment. At night the alcoholic will need more drinks to enable him to sleep. It is not uncommon for an alcoholic to drink a full bottle of spirits in addition to large amounts of wine or beer every day. Drinking is not a pleasure for him, it is an essential part of his life. He gets drunk quickly, and for most of the time feels quite wretched.

Large quantities of drink will eventually have a serious effect on the alcoholic's physical health. Because he prefers drink to food he will suffer from anaemia, vitamin deficiency and be liable

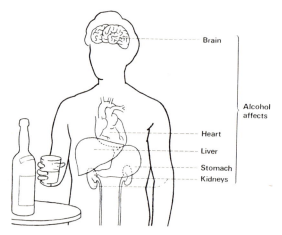

Organs of the body affected by alcohol
Redrawn by courtesy of the Editor, Nursing Times

to chest and other infections. Alcohol will poison his body and may cause peripheral neuritis (inflammation of the nerve endings), gastritis (inflammation of the stomach), cirrhosis of the liver, heart and kidney disorders. Many of these diseases can be fatal if the alcoholic does not stop drinking permanently.

Mentally, the alcoholic can deteriorate seriously. He may suffer from memory loss, become untidy and careless, and be eventually unable to work. Bouts of anger, depression, and even paranoid feelings are not uncommon. Frequently he will say that he is giving up drink, but he never does.

It is very difficult for an alcoholic to remain employed, especially if his job is skilled. He may well be dismissed for continual lateness, drunkenness or incompetence. His family will suffer financially, as most of his income, including the housekeeping money, is spent on drink. Some alcoholics have even mortgaged their houses having spent their own, and other people's money on alcohol. The more fortunate of them remain protected by kindly friends and relations. Others are abandoned, penniless, and eventually forced to live on the streets.

Delirium tremens is an acute mental condition which is common in alcoholics. It frequently occurs after a heavy or prolonged drinking bout. The patient is delirious (see p. 103) and has a tremor of the tongue, lips and hands. The treatment is similar to that of delirium (see p. 103) and the patient is given vitamin B complex by intramuscular or intravenous injection.

Korsakov's psychosis is a serious mental condition which may occur in alcoholics. The symptoms are similar to those of chronic confusion (see p. 105) and the patient tries to conceal his memory loss by making up fantastic stories (confabulation).

Treatment
For treatment to be successful the patient must genuinely want to be cured. He must accept that after treatment he can never again drink alcohol. Weaning the patient from the drug is not difficult. However, it may be extremely hard for him to resist the temptation to start drinking again later.

The patient is best admitted to hospital for treatment, or to a special unit for alcoholics. 'Drying out' is begun as soon as possible. He will usually be prescribed tranquillizing and sedative drugs to help him over the period of withdrawal. Many doctors give large doses of vitamin B complex as a matter of course. During withdrawal the patient will require a great deal of encouragement. He will also need to be supervised to ensure that he does not obtain alcohol.

Antabuse (disulfiram) is a drug commonly used to prevent the patient from drinking alcohol after the period of withdrawal. The drug causes no ill effects unless the patient takes an alcoholic drink. Then he will develop extremely unpleasant symptoms which include a feeling of constriction in the throat, palpitations, nausea and vomiting. Usually the patient is given antabuse for a few days, and then a small amount of alcohol under medical supervision. This demonstrates to the patient the effects of drinking while taking the drug. Unfortunately many patients stop taking antabuse and resume drinking. The other important treatment for alcoholism is aversion therapy. This is discussed in Chapter 16.

After hospital treatment the alcoholic will need continued support from relatives and friends. They should be told that he must never drink again, and that they can best help him by not drinking alcohol in his presence. Alcohol should not be kept indoors. It is often helpful if a close relative gives up drinking as an example to the patient. The alcoholic himself must avoid parties and celebrations, at least until he is confident of his ability to refuse drinks. Alcoholics who experience great difficulty, can perhaps be helped by the organisation called Alcoholics Anonymous (A.A.). Run by ex-alcoholics, A.A. lends support and offers practical advice to people with drink problems. The address and telephone number of Alcoholics Anonymous can be found in most telephone directories.

CASE ILLUSTRATION 14: CHRONIC ALCOHOLISM

'Don't worry, it's only Mrs Norris,' said the staff nurse. The pupil nurse sat back in her chair under the dim light of the observation area. 'You are going to work on this ward for the next three nights I see – you'll get used to Mrs Norris. She gets out of bed several times during the night to go to the toilet. She doesn't like to ask for help, she's a very independent lady. She is a little unsteady when she walks though, so it pays to keep an eye on her.' 'Is she the lady who . . . ?' 'Yes, she's the alcoholic,' answered the staff nurse almost before the question was asked. 'A very nice lady; always so polite and helpful to the other patients too. It certainly disproves the idea that all alcoholics are selfish and rude. It's a shame she drinks like that. She showed me some photographs of herself last night; they were taken a few years ago. She was very pretty then. To look at her now you would not believe she was the same person.' 'What made her start drinking?' asked the pupil nurse, impressed by her colleague's kindly attitude towards Mrs Norris. 'I'm not sure, she was only admitted three days ago. Dr Roberts interviewed her husband this afternoon, so he will have made some notes. Look, the ward is very quiet just now. Why don't you go and take a look through her case notes? You'll find them in the cabinet in the charge nurse's office.'

Mrs Vivian Norris, aged fifty-three years, was admitted at the request of her G.P. after another long drinking bout. She was reported to be drinking a large bottle of gin and a bottle of sherry every day for the past twelve weeks. Her husband noticed that she was having difficulty in breathing a fortnight ago, and says that she seems to be forgetting things that have happened most recently.

This is her first admission here. She has been treated in an alcoholic unit, and later in a nursing home run by a religious order. Her history of drinking is of twenty years' duration. Until five years ago she was employed as a secretary by the G.P.O., when she was dismissed for returning from lunch drunk on several occasions. A few weeks later, she was persuaded to go to the alcoholic unit for treatment, where she stayed for three months. Her husband says that she liked the unit, and during her stay never had a single drink. She was discharged home, and prescribed Antabuse, one tablet three times daily.

Her husband states that she was never very happy at home. They occupied the top flat of a large terraced house; her mother-in-law living downstairs. Her problem seems to be that she has too much time on her hands. There are no children to look after, and her husband works late hours. The situation is not improved by her mother-in-law, who is always criticising her and feels that her son is not being looked after properly. Rows often develop between them, and sometimes between the three of them in the middle of the night. It was after one such row that Mrs

Norris started to drink again, and gave up taking her Antabuse. She drank heavily again for almost a year, and in desperation her husband made private arrangements for her to spend time in a home run by nursing sisters. In the home she stopped drinking once again without difficulty. She was friendly and helpful to the sisters and the other patients, and it was only with some difficulty that the doctor managed to persuade her to leave.

Less than three months after her return home, Mrs Norris started drinking again. This time she would drink in the early morning, and continue all day. Night after night her husband returned home to find her completely drunk. One night he came home from work to find her lying on the floor, her head covered with blood. She had got drunk, fallen into the fire and badly burned her head and cut her face. Being unable to rouse her, Mr Norris immediately called for an ambulance, and she was taken to the accident and emergency department of the local general hospital. The next day she was transferred to the burns unit of a London hospital.

She spent six months in hospital, where she underwent repeated operations for skin grafts to her scalp. Routine investigations in hospital indicated that she had developed cirrhosis of the liver. The consultant told her husband that unless she stopped drinking she would be likely to die within a very short time. Mrs Norris was discharged home, although she kept regular appointments at the out-patients department of the hospital. Her head was so badly burned that the hair roots were damaged, and her hair grew only in patches. Mr Norris bought her an expensive wig, which she insisted was nothing like her real hair.

After a few weeks at home Mrs Norris began drinking heavily again. Her husband tried to persuade her to go into hospital again for treatment, but she constantly refused. Her drinking bouts would last for two or three months at a time, when she would suddenly announce that she had given up for good. The pride she once took in her house and personal appearance began to decline, and it was during the last drinking bout that she refused to cook and clean the house, and spent all day in bed. During the day she would get up to go to the toilet, and in the evenings she would dress and walk to the off licence for fresh supplies of gin and sherry. She would often complain of pains in her arms and legs, and remarked that she was becoming too fat.

Mr Norris sent for her G.P. two weeks ago when he noticed that his wife was gasping for breath. The doctor arrived to find her lying in bed drinking heavily from the large bottle of gin on the bedside table. She begged the doctor not to take her drink away, and appealed to him to arrange for her to go to hospital.

On admission she was examined by the duty doctor, and arrangements were made for her to have a blood analysis, and an electrocardiogram at the local general hospital. He prescribed aminophylline, 100 mg three times daily to help ease her breathing, and frusemide, 40 mg in the mornings to help reduce the oedema in her legs and feet.

The pupil nurse turned to the nurses' notes at the back of the case folder, and read yesterday's entry. 'Mrs Norris has settled in well, and apparently is not craving for alcohol. She says she is glad to be here so that we can help her to stop drinking. Despite her poor physical condition she insists on getting up early in the day to help with the ward work. She appears to enjoy the ward meetings, and tries to help the other patients. She has asked if she can be allowed to go for a ride in her husband's car when he comes to visit her tomorrow.'

'Well, we had better make a final round before we go off duty,' said the staff nurse. 'The day staff will be here in half an hour, and I have to complete the report.' 'Yes, it's been a long night; no problems and so very quiet,' replied the pupil. 'You'll see that it isn't always like this,' and both nurses walked down the corridor to take a look at the patients in each room. 'Mrs Norris! Mrs Norris!' the staff nurse heard the raised voice of her colleague and ran into the side room. She quickly felt for the patient's pulse, but there was none. 'Quick, nurse, telephone the doctor and ask him to get here immediately!' The staff nurse removed the pillow from behind her patient's head.

It was almost 8.30 a.m. before the staff nurse began to write the final report. 'Have you informed Mr Norris?' asked the charge nurse. 'Yes, the nursing officer telephoned the police just before

8 o'clock. He will probably be along soon.' 'Do the other patients know? They are going to be upset about this. They all thought Mrs Norris was a kind, polite lady.'

The result of the inquest, held just a week later, was that Mrs Norris died from cardiac failure. The pathologist stated that she had probably been dead only a short time before she was found. He gave evidence that she had cirrhosis of the liver, renal damage and coronary thrombosis. Probably out of kindness to Mr Norris, no mention was made in court of the true cause of his wife's death.

QUESTIONS

1 Name four drugs which are frequently misused.
*2 Name two effects which amphetamines have on the body.
3 What do you understand by the term 'drug addiction'?
4 Give two reasons why a person may become addicted to drugs.
5 What do you understand by the term 'withdrawal symptoms'?
6 Name three physical illnesses which may be caused by drinking alcohol excessively.
7 Mention one treatment for alcoholism.

* Reproduced by permission of The General Nursing Council for England and Wales.

Chapter 11

EPILEPSY

Epilepsy is the name given to sudden losses of consciousness which are often accompanied by repeated jerking movements called **convulsions**. These attacks are sometimes called **fits** or **seizures**. Epilepsy is not a mental illness, but occasionally an epileptic patient can benefit from treatment in a psychiatric hospital.

CAUSES

The brain is made up of millions of cells, each cell producing a small electrical discharge. Normally the electrical activity of the brain is regulated, but in some people uncontrolled discharges suddenly occur, causing an epileptic fit. Exactly why this should happen is not known.

Epilepsy frequently begins in childhood, and very often no cause can be found. Epilepsy which has no known physical or other cause is called **primary** or **idiopathic** epilepsy. Primary epilepsy is more common among children of low intelligence, and in some cases it is inherited.

When a cause of epileptic fits is known, the condition is called **secondary** or **symptomatic** epilepsy. Secondary epilepsy may occur at any time of life and can be caused by a number of diseases of the brain or body. Some common causes are:

Congenital brain disease
Injury of the brain at birth or later in life
Brain tumour
Infection of the brain, e.g. with syphilis
Senile dementia and pre-senile dementia
Poisoning, especially with alcohol or carbon monoxide
The toxic effect of renal failure
The side effects of some drugs.

TYPES OF FIT

There are several types of epileptic fit. Some patients may only experience one type, while others may have several different types of fit.

MAJOR FIT

This type of seizure can be very frightening to onlookers, particularly if they have not seen an epileptic fit before. The stages of a major fit are:

1   The **aura** which sometimes warns the patient that he is going to have a seizure. He may feel a strange sensation in his stomach, hear an unusual noise, or sense that something odd is about to happen. Sometimes a patient may experience a certain taste or smell just before the fit.

2   The **tonic** stage follows the aura, when the patient suddenly becomes unconscious. If he is standing he will fall to the ground. He may give a short cry as he falls. His muscles go into spasm and his limbs are stretched out rigidly in front of him. His eyes are rolled upwards, his jaw is tightly shut, and he stops breathing. The tonic stage lasts for about thirty seconds.

3   The **clonic** stage follows immediately. Although the patient remains unconscious, his muscles start to relax and contract alternately. His head, body and limbs jerk repeatedly, and he starts to breathe again. Quite often his bladder will be emptied. The clonic stage lasts for one to three minutes.

4   **Recovery** follows gradually and the patient regains consciousness. Afterwards he may be very confused or complain of severe headache. Sometimes he will feel very tired and may sleep after the fit. Occasionally, a patient may appear to have recovered but walks about unaware of what he is doing. In this state he can easily wander away or attack other people. This type of behaviour is called **post epileptic automatism**.

MINOR FIT

A minor epileptic fit is a short period of unconsciousness. The patient loses consciousness only for a few seconds. He will suddenly stop whatever he is doing, and if he is holding something he may drop it. He will stare vacantly for a short time, but hardly ever falls to the ground. There are no convulsions, but sometimes his face may twitch slightly. When the patient recovers, he is able to carry on with whatever he was doing.

JACKSONIAN EPILEPSY

This type of fit begins in one part of the body and can spread to other parts. For example, the seizure can start in the patient's thumb and spread to his hand, arm and face. Sometimes the fit spreads all over the body becoming a major epileptic fit.

STATUS EPILEPTICUS

Occasionally a patient may have a series of major fits, one after the other, without regaining consciousness in between. This is called status epilepticus. The condition can last for about half an hour, but sometimes it continues for several days with the patient having hundreds of fits. Status epilepticus sometimes occurs when the patient does not take his drugs regularly, or during a physical illness. It is an extremely dangerous condition as he can easily die from heart failure or pneumonia, and must be treated by a doctor urgently.

TEMPORAL LOBE EPILEPSY

When the electrical discharges which usually cause seizures arise in the temporal lobes of the brain only, the condition is called temporal lobe epilepsy. The patient does not have a convulsion but enters a dream-like state, and he may have frightening visions or hear strange voices. Sometimes, he is very confused and may attack other people. When he recovers from the attack he will not be able to remember very well what has happened. Quite naturally, he will be very frightened that it may occur again.

EPILEPSY AND MENTAL ILLNESS

Most people who suffer from epilepsy never need to be treated in a psychiatric hospital. However, like other people, epileptics can become mentally ill. Occasionally an epileptic patient is admitted to hospital because his behaviour can no longer be tolerated. He may become irritable, or even paranoid and hostile. Chronic epileptics are sometimes slow and clumsy in the way they move, and may become seriously confused at times. Often they find difficulty in putting their thoughts together, and may take a long time to explain what they mean. Young epileptic patients often have temper tantrums, and their relatives may find it impossible to care for them.

Sometimes the epileptic patient's abnormal behaviour is a result of his frequent fits. However, the difficulties and frustration he will have experienced in life must also have an effect on him. As a child he may have been over-protected by his parents. At school he will have been different from the others, unable to join in many of their activities. Almost certainly he will have found great difficulty in finding a job, or in keeping one. For these reasons he may feel resentful and suspicious, and behave in an unacceptable way.

TREATMENT DURING A FIT

MAJOR FIT

If the patient has an aura, and is able to tell the nurse, he should be helped to lie down on his bed. Very often he will lose consciousness suddenly without having time to warn anyone. If possible he should be caught before he falls down and put gently on to the floor. If he falls to the ground he should only be moved if he is in danger of hurting himself.

When the patient is on the floor the nurse should loosen his collar and place a cushion under his head. During the tonic stage of the fit no attempt should be made to force anything between his teeth. When the clonic stage begins it may be possible to place a rubber mouth gag or folded handkerchief between his teeth to stop him biting his tongue. His movements should not be restrained unless he is in danger of hurting himself.

A nurse must stay with the patient during all stages of an epileptic fit. When he has regained consciousness she should examine him for injuries. He should be allowed to rest on the floor for a short time and then helped to his bed or to an armchair. If the patient has been incontinent, the nurse should take him to the bathroom and provide him with a change of clothes. If he wants to sleep after the fit he should be allowed to do so, and if he is confused, or is known to suffer from post epileptic automatism, a nurse must remain with him until he is fully recovered. A written report of the fit must be made as soon as possible.

MINOR FIT

There is no special treatment for a minor fit. If the patient feels unwell or is surprised at the attack, the nurse should reassure him. A written report must be made of the fit.

JACKSONIAN EPILEPSY

If the fit is mild no special treatment is required. The nurse should remain with the patient and observe him carefully. A detailed, written report of the seizure should be made immediately afterwards. The report must state where on the body the convulsions started, and exactly where they spread. This information is essential to the doctor who is treating the patient.

STATUS EPILEPTICUS

This is a very dangerous condition as the patient may die without medical attention. A doctor must be informed immediately a patient has two or more fits without recovering consciousness in between. Meanwhile, the nurse must ensure that he has a clear airway, using suction apparatus if necessary to remove mucous from his mouth and pharynx. The doctor will prescribe **anticonvulsant** drugs to be given by intravenous or intramuscular injection. Until he recovers, the nursing care is that given to all

unconscious patients. His pressure areas must be treated, and his
position in bed changed frequently. The doctor may decide that
he should be tube fed or given an intravenous infusion. If the fits
continue, the patient may be sent to an intensive care unit in a
general hospital.

TEMPORAL LOBE EPILEPSY

During the attack the patient will need to be closely observed.
He must not be allowed to wander away from the ward. If his
behaviour is violent, several nurses should be available to prevent
injury (see violent behaviour, p. 161). The patient may be very
frightened after he has recovered, and the nurse should be prepared to reassure him.

TREATMENT OF EPILEPSY

Epilepsy can be investigated by a special test called an electroencephalogram (E.E.G.). Small electrodes are placed on the
patient's head, and the wires leading from them are plugged into
a recording machine. The tiny electric currents given off by the
brain are amplified and recorded on paper. Specialists are often
able to tell from the recording what type of epilepsy the patient
has. The E.E.G. investigation is not painful, as electricity is not
passed through the patient's brain.

Epilepsy is treated by **anticonvulsant** drugs. They help to
control the frequency and severity of the patient's fits. The drugs
must be taken regularly, as missing a dose may cause him to have
a series of fits. Examples of anticonvulsant drugs are sulthiame,
phenytoin sodium, primidone and phenobarbitone. Anticonvulsants, like most other drugs, sometimes cause symptoms
known as **side effects**. The common side effects of anticonvulsant drugs are:

confusion	nausea and vomiting
drowsiness	skin rashes
giddiness	tenderness of the gums

If any of these symptoms occur a doctor must be informed immediately.

Occasionally, an epileptic patient will stop having fits completely after drug therapy. However, most will need to take anticonvulsants indefinitely. Sometimes, a patient may benefit from brain surgery.

GENERAL MANAGEMENT

In the past, people often believed that those who suffered from epileptic fits were possessed by the Devil. Epileptics were given the most crude forms of medical treatment or subjected to torture. Unfortunately, even today, some of the superstition which surrounded epilepsy still remains. People who witness an epileptic fit quite often become afraid, and epileptic patients find themselves rejected by other members of society.

A child who suffers from epilepsy is at a disadvantage from the start. He feels different from other children because he cannot join in many of their games. If he has fits in the classroom he may be rejected or ridiculed by them. He can easily fall behind with his school work, or if he has frequent fits, he may be sent to a special school.

An epileptic person will find difficulty in getting a job or in keeping one. Very often employers will dismiss someone who has fits, and employees are reluctant to work with epileptics. Of course there are many jobs which an epileptic should not do. He must not work with moving machinery, climb ladders, drive motor vehicles or work at any job where sudden unconsciousness could be dangerous. It is not surprising, in view of all their frustrations, that epileptics can become difficult, hostile people.

As with any other illness which is unlikely to be cured, epilepsy must be accepted by the patient if he is not to become embittered and helpless. Some restrictions are inevitable and have to be accepted; other problems can be overcome with help and understanding from those who care for him. Accepting the disability may be a slow process. In hospital it is more likely to be achieved if the patient is encouraged to do things for himself, and if restrictions are kept to a minimum.

When an epileptic patient is admitted to a psychiatric hospital, the nursing and medical staff should decide together the best way of caring for him. They must take into account his age, behaviour and the frequency of his fits when deciding upon restrictions and supervision. Sometimes it is worth taking small risks if the patient will benefit from greater freedom and independence.

A general rule when caring for an epileptic patient is to protect him from the worst dangers, but not in a way that will make him feel helpless and restricted. One patient may need close observation when bathing, eating or making tea; another will need only limited supervision. Attention to small but important details can make life more comfortable for the patient and protect him from obvious dangers. He should be provided with a fairly hard pillow for his bed. He must be told to inform the nurse before he takes a bath, and advised not to fill the bath too full. If the patient can see the real need for the precautions he is more likely to accept them without resentment.

It cannot be denied that some epileptic patients are difficult to nurse. Their resentment, hostility and suspicion can present real problems to those who care for them. With kindness, tact and genuine interest in their welfare, it is possible to overcome these difficulties and gain their trust.

QUESTIONS

1 What do you understand by the term 'idiopathic epilepsy'?
2 Give three causes of symptomatic epilepsy.
3 List the stages of a major epileptic fit.
4 What do you understand by the term 'post-epileptic automatism'?
5 What is meant by the term 'status epilepticus'?
6 Name two drugs used in the treatment of epilepsy.
7 Give three side effects of anticonvulsant drugs.
8 Mention two common problems of epileptic people in the community.
9 Mention two difficulties of nursing long-stay epileptic patients.

10 What do you understand by the term 'Jacksonian epilepsy'?

11 What precautions would you take when giving an epileptic patient a bath?

*12 What occupations are not suitable for epileptic patients?

* Reproduced by permission of The General Nursing Council for England and Wales.

Chapter 12

MENTAL SUBNORMALITY

Mental subnormality is a state of arrested or incomplete development of the mind which requires special care or treatment. People who are mentally subnormal have not developed the intelligence and abilities which we take for granted. Intelligence is the capacity to deal with new information, situations and ideas. It enables us to learn, and apply what we have learned in a way that is meaningful. A person who lacks intelligence will clearly encounter many difficulties in life. Some people are so mentally subnormal and lacking in intelligence that they are unable to lead normal, everyday lives. They have to be looked after by relatives or admitted to special institutions.

Mental subnormality is diagnosed during the first few years of a child's life. The doctor or midwife who is present at the birth of the baby may observe appearances which indicate that he is mentally subnormal. Often the health visitor or doctor at the infant welfare clinic will observe that his development is delayed. Occasionally this passes un-noticed until the child goes to school, when his school teacher may notice that something is wrong.

Whenever the condition is first noticed, the child will be sent with his parents to a special assessment clinic. There he will be examined by a specialist who is able to decide the best form of treatment and give advice to his parents.

CAUSES

There are many causes of mental subnormality. Some of the most common are:

1 *Genetic.* The condition may be passed from parents to child by the genes. Usually the parents are quite normal, and it is impossible to tell that they stand a chance of producing a subnormal child.

2 *Damage before birth.* Certain conditions which affect the pregnant mother can also damage the unborn child, e.g. if she has German measles during the first three months of pregnancy, syphilis, or is exposed to X-rays.

3 *Damage during birth.* The baby's brain may be damaged during birth by forceps or lack of oxygen.

4 *Damage after birth.* The child may have a disease which can hinder mental development, e.g. meningitis. Head injury, brain tumour and poisoning with lead can also cause mental subnormality.

SUBNORMALITY AND SEVERE SUBNORMALITY

People who are mentally subnormal can be divided into two groups, the subnormal and the severely subnormal.

SUBNORMAL PEOPLE

Their level of intelligence and abilities are varied. However, they are always below average, but at a higher level than those of the severely subnormal. What they are able to do depends upon the degree of subnormality and the type of care and training they have received. Most subnormal people will be able to hold a simple conversation, or at least use short sentences. Many of them will be able to tell the time, read a few words, and write their name. They will not be able to tackle skilled or complex tasks, although they may be quite happy doing simple jobs such as washing up, cleaning or labouring. It will be very difficult for them to follow complicated instructions or absorb a lot of information at one time.

Subnormal people find great difficulty in learning, and will not achieve very much at school. Some of them will find very simple jobs which they will do eagerly for the rest of their lives. Others are unreliable and cannot keep a job for more than a few weeks at a time. If a subnormal person marries, it is generally to someone of similar ability. Without guidance they may have too many children and find themselves unable to cope.

Many subnormal people are able to live in the community and get by, despite difficulties. Others can manage with a great deal of support from relatives and the social services. Some have to be admitted to hospital because they can no longer deal with problems, or become too great a burden on other people.

SEVERELY SUBNORMAL PEOPLE

Their intelligence and abilities are lower than those of the subnormal. Even with care and training they will always be dependent on other people. If left to fend for themselves they are in danger of being exploited by others.

Some severely subnormal people can use simple language, learn to write a few words, and recognise objects. A few can be taught to do simple tasks, but their understanding is very limited. Others are unable to master even basic skills, and have to be washed, fed and taken to the lavatory. Many are incontinent, unable to walk and need constant nursing care. A few have outbursts of destructiveness and noisiness for no apparent reason.

Severely subnormal people often have serious physical disabilities which restrict them even further. They may be physically underdeveloped, and often appear ugly. Their heads are sometimes too large or too small, or mis-shapen. They may have slanting eyes or a tongue which is too large. Some suffer from blindness, deafness, heart disease, epilepsy or paralysis. A few are so phycially disabled that they have to be nursed in bed. Some severely subnormal children die in the first few years of life, usually from heart disease or chest infections.

SPECIAL TYPES OF MENTAL SUBNORMALITY

Some people who are mentally subnormal can be recognised as suffering from special conditions. Some of the more common of these are:

MONGOLISM (DOWN'S DISEASE)

Mongolism is caused by an inherited abnormality of the chromosomes in the child's cells. Mongol children are often born to mothers who are approaching middle age, but why this is so is not known.

The condition is called Mongolism because the children look something like the people of Mongolia. All Mongol children look very much alike. A typical child has a small, round head, broad nose and slanting eyes. His tongue is too large and protrudes from his mouth. He will be shorter than a normal child for his age, and has a tendency to become fat. Most mongol children are severely subnormal and many have abnormalities of the heart.

PHENYLKETONURIA

This is an inherited disease of the child's metabolism. A particular protein cannot be dealt with properly by the body; it remains in the bloodstream and prevents normal mental development. Most white children who suffer from this condition have fair hair and blue eyes. If they are not diagnosed and treated soon after birth they will become severely subnormal.

The condition can be discovered by a special blood test. All babies are tested for it shortly after birth. Treatment is to reduce the amount of harmful protein by giving the child a special diet until he reaches adulthood.

CRETINISM

This condition is caused by a congenital defect of the thyroid gland. It is usually discovered when the baby is a few months old. His mother will notice that he sleeps a lot, cries very little and is not interested in feeding. If he is not treated he will be mentally retarded and physically under-developed.

The treatment for cretinism is by giving the child thyroid extract. If the condition is discovered early enough and treated, he will develop quite normally.

MICROCEPHALUS

Microcephalus means small head. The size and shape of the child's head is very noticeable. His forehead slopes backwards sharply, and his scalp lies in folds over his skull. Most of these children are severely subnormal. Microcephalus can be inherited, or it can be caused by the mother having German measles during the first three months of pregnancy.

HYDROCEPHALUS

In this condition the circulation of the fluid in the brain (cerebro-spinal fluid) is obstructed. This causes damage to the brain and enlargement of the skull. It may be an inherited abnormality or a complication of meningitis in early childhood.

A few of these babies are born with enlarged heads, but most develop the condition after birth. The skull becomes larger and larger, and in time the child may not be able to lift his head from his pillow. He may become blind, paralysed and suffer from epileptic fits. All children who suffer from hydrocephalus are subnormal or severely subnormal. Many die in early childhood. The condition can sometimes be relieved by the operation of inserting a valve which allows the fluid to drain into the blood-stream. The operation is a complicated one, and very often the valve becomes blocked after a short while.

LEAD POISONING

Lead poisoning in children can cause mental subnormality, epileptic fits, blindness and paralysis. A child may poison himself accidentally by sucking toys, eating paint or chewing objects containing lead. For this reason the sale of toys which contain lead is against the law in the United Kingdom.

TREATMENT IN THE COMMUNITY

It is a great shock for parents to be told that their child is mentally subnormal. Some parents cannot accept at first that he will never be like other children. They may take him from one specialist to another until they finally come to terms with the truth. Other parents start to blame themselves or each other, and feel in some way responsible for their child's condition. In the end, parents generally accept the fact and insist that they look after the child at home.

It is much better for the child if he can be cared for at home rather than sent to an institution. However, this can produce many problems for the whole family. Neighbours may gossip about them and keep their own children away from the subnormal child. Many people still hold the mistaken belief that having a subnormal child is punishment for the parents' wickedness. Other children too can be very cruel. They are always ready to play tricks on the subnormal child and poke fun at him. In addition to these problems, caring for the child is a great responsibility for his parents. Normal children quickly achieve a measure of independence. They go to school, mix with other children, and need less and less supervision as time goes by. The subnormal child may need constant care and protection. He may never go to a normal school. He will grow up physically, but in mind he will always remain childish. In spite of all the problems, parents generally become devoted to their subnormal child, and would not dream of sending him to an institution.

In caring for their child, parents can be helped by social workers and other services provided by the local authority. It is often possible for him to be sent to hospital or a residential home for a few weeks while his parents take a holiday. When he is old enough to go to school, the child may be sent to a special school for the educationally subnormal (E.S.N. school), or a school for the severely subnormal (S.S.N. school). There he will be helped by specially trained teachers to read, write and develop to the best of his ability. Children who cannot benefit from an E.S.N. or S.S.N. school because their mental and physical handicap is so severe, can be sent to a local **special care unit**.

When the child leaves school, the local authority may be able to help find him a simple job at which he can earn a living. If he is unable to work, a place may be found for him in an Adult Training Centre. Here he can learn skills to prepare him for a job in the community. Many local authorities provide sheltered workshops for young adults who are unable to do a regular, productive job. Local authority **hostels** provide sheltered living accommodation for adults who are unable to live at home, but who need some care and supervision. All of these important services need to be improved and extended. Only in this way can parents of subnormal children be relieved of their most serious worry – 'What happens when we can no longer look after him?'

TREATMENT IN HOSPITAL

Some mentally subnormal children cannot be cared for at home. It may be that the child places an intolerable strain on the family, or is so physically disabled that hospital care is the only answer. Some older children and adults are admitted because their behaviour is no longer acceptable. Occasionally, very young babies are rejected by their parents and have to be sent to hospital.

Throughout the United Kingdom there are hospitals which specialise in the treatment of the mentally subnormal. The aim of treatment is to train the child to become as independent as possible. Some children are eventually able to leave hospital. Others will need to be looked after for the rest of their lives.

On admission to hospital the child is given a thorough physical and mental examination. The hospital team will assess his physical and mental capabilities and decide on a policy for his care and training. Some severely subnormal children are so physically disabled that they have to be nursed in bed. In such cases specialised nursing care is the most important part of treatment. Others who are capable of greater development will first of all be trained to walk, go to the toilet and eat without assistance.

When he is old enough the more able child will be sent to the hospital school. Like a normal child, but more slowly, he will learn through play and activity. Specially trained teachers will help him to talk, recognise objects and even to read and count a little.

The older hospital patient, if he is capable, will be trained for some kind of work. Facilities exist for teaching domestic work, laundry work or simple factory and production line jobs. If it is thought that a patient will eventually be able to work and live outside hospital, he will be taught to live independently. Most hospitals have small flats or houses where patients can live and learn to look after themselves. When he finds a job he will be allowed to live in the hospital for some time until he is able to care for himself with the minimum of supervision.

For the patient who must remain in hospital permanently, much can be done to make his life comfortable. Relatives will be encouraged to visit him as much as possible, and even to take him home for week-ends and holidays. The hospital provides entertainments such as film shows, parties and socials. There will be shopping trips, visits to the country, the theatre and other places of interest. Many hospitals have holiday homes at the seaside where patients can spend time in the summer. Other hospitals organise seaside holidays in hotels, or even supervised trips abroad.

The mentally subnormal cannot be cured. However, with adequate facilities many of these unfortunate people can be helped to develop what capacities they have to the full, and to lead more useful, happier lives. Much has been done in recent years to improve conditions for them in hospital and in the community. It is to be hoped that this trend will continue in the future.

QUESTIONS

1   What do you understand by the term 'mental subnormality'?
2   Mention three causes of mental subnormality.
3   Name three disorders associated with mental subnormality.
4   State two problems of caring for a mentally subnormal child at home.
5   Mention three facilities provided to help the mentally subnormal person in the community.
6   State one aim of nursing subnormal patients in hospital.

Chapter 13

FRINGE PROBLEMS

In a psychiatric hospital there are patients who are not truly mentally ill, but who have problems of one sort or another. Sometimes people other than psychiatrists, such as physicians, social workers and ministers of religion are able to deal with these problems. Often a psychiatrist may be asked to help because he is considered best able to handle a particular difficulty. Some of the more common problems of the 'fringes' of psychiatry are discussed here.

PSYCHOSOMATIC DISORDERS

The word psychosomatic means mind and body. Psychosomatic disorders are conditions in which emotional disturbances play a large part in producing physical symptoms. Just as the emotion of anxiety can produce sweating, palpitations and tremor (see Anxiety Neurosis p. 58), so emotions can help to cause more serious illnesses. Many of these serious conditions are treated in a general hospital rather than in a hospital for the mentally ill. Even so, many doctors consider the psychological aspects of the illnesses to be very important, and prescribe treatment accordingly. For this reason some of the conditions which are often regarded as psychosomatic are discussed here.

ANOREXIA NERVOSA

Anorexia nervosa is a condition in which the patient's appetite is lost. The illness usually affects adolescent girls, and there is a serious risk of death from undernourishment. There is no known cause of the condition, but most of the patients have emotional problems. Because of these emotional difficulties many anorexic patients are admitted to a psychiatric hospital for treatment at some stage of the illness.

A girl suffering from anorexia nervosa will look pale and drawn, and will be grossly underweight. Some patients weigh 39 kg (6 stones) or less. She may have a covering of fine hair on her limbs, and menstruation will have ceased. Despite her severe weight loss she will say that she is getting fat, and will constantly refuse food. Indeed, she may insist on taking regular exercise, and purge herself with laxatives, to help her lose even more weight.

The treatment for anorexia nervosa is to ensure that the girl takes adequate, regular meals and regains weight. She must then eat enough to maintain the average weight for her height. All this is easier said than done. Persuading an anorexic patient to eat can be one of the most difficult problems a nurse will encounter.

Generally the girl is put to bed after admission to hospital. She must be encouraged to take regular, attractive meals. The nurse should insist gently, but firmly that the meal must be eaten, and should never argue or bargain with her. Once the patient has eaten the first meal it will be much easier to persuade her to eat again. However, she must never be left alone while eating, and should be observed for some time after the meal. Patients suffering from anorexia nervosa are past-masters at hiding food, and some of them will vomit deliberately after eating. A careful record of the patient's weight must always be kept, and it is helpful if a written note is made of each meal taken.

If the patient cannot be persuaded to eat, the doctor will give permission for her to be tube fed. Tube feeding must be carried out gently but firmly, and discontinued as soon as she is willing to eat. Sometimes the doctor may feel that tranquillizing drugs such as diazepam or chlorpromazine may help the patient. Often she will be asked to attend group or individual psychotherapy sessions with a psychiatrist or psychologist.

When the patient has regained sufficient weight and is eating regularly, she will be discharged from hospital. An appointment will be made for her at the outpatient's clinic where her weight will be checked regularly. Fortunately, most anorexic patients recover completely, although a few may need to be re-admitted to hospital from time to time.

PEPTIC ULCER

A peptic ulcer is caused by the gastric juice digesting an area of the wall of the stomach or duodenum. The condition is extremely painful, and occasionally a patient may die from internal haemorrhage or other complications. Peptic ulcers frequently occur in people who constantly worry. Businessmen and hard working, ambitious people are also prone to them.

A patient with a peptic ulcer is always treated at a general hospital. Often the condition can be cured by drugs and a special diet, but sometimes surgical treatment is necessary. Frequently the physician will prescribe tranquillizing drugs for the patient, to combat stress and anxiety.

ULCERATIVE COLITIS

Ulcerative colitis is a disease of the large intestine. The colon becomes inflamed, and the patient suffers from diarrhoea, bleeding and severe abdominal pain. The condition tends to be chronic, and there is a danger that the patient may die.

There is no known cause of ulcerative colitis. The disease sometimes follows an emotional upset such as a broken love affair or death of a loved one. It is generally treated medically with drugs and a special diet, but sometimes an operation to remove part of the colon is carried out.

OBESITY

Obesity is a store of excess fat in the tissues of the body. The most common cause of obesity is overeating. Fat people easily develop heart and respiratory diseases, and disorders of the digestive tract. Despite these dangers, many people continually eat excessive amounts of food. They often want to lose weight, but find that overeating is a habit which they cannot break.

Emotional problems are frequently a cause of overeating. Some obese people eat when they are anxious because it helps to relieve their tension. Others eat when they are miserable and find consolation in food. For these patients, psychotherapy may be of great benefit in helping them to lose weight. Psychotherapy sessions may be held in hospitals, weight clinics and private slimming clubs. Some patients may be prescribed drugs to help curb appetite, and a low calorie diet is always necessary.

ASTHMA

Asthma is really difficulty in breathing characterised by wheezing. An attack of asthma can last from a few minutes to several days. It can be very distressing for the patient, who has to fight for his breath and may feel that he is going to suffocate.

An attack of asthma occurs when the small bronchial muscles contract and the mucous membranes of the lungs swell. It is not known exactly why this happens. Some patients appear to be sensitive to pollens, dust and other particles in the air. However, attacks often occur when the patient is under stress. Many asthma sufferers are anxious, moody and dependent people.

A severe attack of asthma is often treated with injections of adrenaline or aminophylline. The patient should be propped up in a position which makes it easier for him to breathe. A person who suffers from repeated attacks may be prescribed tablets of ephedrine or special inhalants, and is usually encouraged to take regular breathing exercises.

SEXUAL PROBLEMS

When a person is unable to achieve satisfaction through normal sexual intercourse he may have a sexual problem. Sexual activity only becomes a problem to a person if it causes him, or other people, unhappiness or concern. A large number of people experience sexual difficulties at least for a short time during their lives. Many are able to resolve them without advice from specialists. A few are less fortunate and need professional help to overcome their problems. Some of the more common sexual problems are discussed here.

IMPOTENCE AND FRIGIDITY

When a man finds difficulty in carrying through sexual inter-course to a climax, the condition is called impotence. It may happen because he is unable to sustain an erection or ejaculates too soon. When a woman is unable to enjoy sexual intercourse and achieve satisfaction from it, the condition is known as frigidity. Both conditions can be caused by anxiety, marital problems or ignorance of sex. Sometimes the problems are caused by childhood experiences, or by a feeling that sex is 'dirty'. Impotence and frigidity may only be temporary. If they continue for any length of time one or both partners should seek help.

HOMOSEXUALITY

Homosexuality means a sexual attraction towards a person of the same sex. There are male and female homosexuals. A woman who is homosexual is sometimes referred to as a lesbian. Some people may be attracted to members of their own sex and the opposite sex, and are called bisexuals.

Research has shown that a large number of people have had some homosexual experience during their lives. Possibly two or three people in every hundred are entirely homosexual. Homosexuality is not a sickness, or a mental illness. It is only a problem if the person is dissatisfied with this part of his life and wishes to change it. Only a few male homosexuals are effeminate, and only a few female homosexuals are masculine. Most of them are quite normal in appearance and in the way in which they behave.

A person who is homosexual may experience many difficulties in life. Homosexuals are often criticised, and may be rejected by their relatives and colleagues. Some are afraid that their position in life will be threatened if the truth is discovered. Despite these problems, many homosexuals are able to achieve a great deal in life and maintain satisfactory personal relationships.

A person who is homosexual may of course become mentally ill and require treatment. Sometimes a person may seek advice from a psychiatrist because of homosexuality itself. Quite often the most a psychiatrist can do is to encourage him to accept his behaviour, and help him deal with his anxiety. Doubtless, help for most homosexuals must come from a greater general understanding and acceptance by society.

PAEDOPHILIA

Paedophilia is a sexual attraction to children. A paedophiliac is generally a man, and he may handle a child sexually or persuade a child to masturbate him. Only very rarely do paedophiliacs cause physical harm to children.

Molesting a child sexually is strictly against the law, and is punished very severely. Paedophiliacs are a problem to society because the well-being of young children is at risk. However, it should not be forgotten that many paedophiliacs are disgusted by their own behaviour, but cannot alter it no matter how hard they try. Many paedophiliacs convicted of an offence are sent to prison. The few who are considered to be in need of treatment may be sent to a psychiatric hospital, often under a Court Order. Although various methods of treatment have been tried, none hold out much hope of success.

TRANSVESTISM

Transvestism is an experience of gaining sexual satisfaction by dressing in clothes of the opposite sex. There are more male than female transvestites, and they are generally not homosexuals. Transvestism only becomes a problem if the person wishes to alter his behaviour, or it upsets other people. Occasionally a transvestite may be admitted to hospital for treatment. An attempt will then be made to help him, often with the use of behaviour therapy (see p. 178).

FETISHISM

Fetishism is a way of gaining sexual satisfaction from objects or articles of clothing, rather than from other people. A few of the people who steal washing no doubt have a fetish for certain articles of clothing. Fetishism does not seem to trouble people very much. In a very minor form it is probably a natural part of human behaviour.

VOYEURISM

Voyeurism is a way of gaining sexual satisfaction from watching other people undress or having sexual intercourse. 'Peeping Toms' are sometimes discovered and fined by the courts. Apart from the annoyance of the people who are being watched, voyeurism does not seem to cause much of a problem. Like fetishism, it is to a certain extent part of normal behaviour.

SADISM

Sadism is a desire to obtain sexual satisfaction by inflicting pain on other people. As long as the sadist's partner is willing to tolerate his behaviour it does not generally become a problem.

MASOCHISM

Masochism is a desire to experience pain at the hands of another person. It is generally not considered to be a great problem, as a masochist is always a willing victim.

CRIME AND MENTAL ILLNESS

There is no mental illness which always makes a person who suffers from it commit a crime. There is also no truth in the belief that all criminals are mentally ill. Most crimes are committed by people who simply believe that they stand to gain some advantage if they are not caught. However, some crimes are committed by people who are mentally ill. Often this is because they are emotionally disturbed or aggressive, or do not realize that they are breaking the law. Mentally ill people who commit crimes are often sent to hospital for treatment. Some of the most common of these crimes are:

PHYSICAL ASSAULT

Most mentally ill people are not violent. Only a few become very disturbed and attack other people. A paranoid person may attack his imagined persecutor because he is very afraid. The person attacked is often a relative, friend or neighbour. A manic patient may become so frustrated and lacking in control that he assaults other people. When a mentally ill person becomes violent the assault is generally not planned. Often it happens because other people start to argue with him or attempt to control his behaviour.

DAMAGE TO PROPERTY

A mentally ill person may try to damage property because he is hallucinated or deluded. He may, for example, see a chair as a wild animal and try to destroy it. A paranoid person, who is convinced that his neighbours are plotting against him, may break the windows of their houses. Sometimes a manic patient who has lost control may try to destroy most of the objects around him.

SHOPLIFTING

Stealing goods from shops and department stores is an extremely common crime. Although most of the people who do it are not considered to be mentally ill, it is interesting that many are carrying enough money to pay for their shopping. Apart from teenagers who raid shops in gangs, most shoplifters are middle aged. Occasionally a shoplifter is discovered to have been extremely anxious or depressed. A confused, elderly person may accidentally take goods without paying for them. A few people steal from shops hoping to get caught, often to embarrass relatives or draw attention to their emotional problems.

SEXUAL OFFENCES

The most common sexual crimes dealt with in hospital are those against young children (see Paedophilia, p. 155). The patient is nearly always detained under a Court Order.

MURDER

Probably the most common form of murder which is caused by mental illness or emotional disturbance is infanticide (child-killing). A mother who kills her young baby is usually depressed or emotionally disturbed. In most cases, the mother is sent to hospital for treatment or placed under psychiatric supervision. A paranoid person may sometimes kill the person he believes to be plotting against him. A depressed person may kill his relatives if he believes that they have a serious illness from which they will eventually die. An epileptic patient may kill someone during a period of post-epileptic automatism without realising what he has done (see Epilepsy, Chapter 11). A psychopathic patient will sometimes kill another person if he cannot get his own way or has been provoked. Nearly all mentally ill people who are convicted of murder are detained in Special Hospitals for reasons of security. There they are treated by psychiatrists and are discharged only when they are considered to be well enough, and with the permission of the Home Secretary. Some patients who have committed murder or other serious crimes may be sent after a time in a Special Hospital, to an ordinary psychiatric hospital, where their treatment can continue.

QUESTIONS

1 What do you understand by the term 'psychosomatic disorder'?
2 Mention two illnesses which are often regarded as psychosomatic.
3 Give two reasons why a patient with a sexual problem may need help from a psychiatrist.
4 State three reasons why a mentally ill person may commit a crime.
5 Give one reason why a mentally ill person may try to destroy property.
6 What is the main function of a Special Hospital?

Chapter 14

AGGRESSIVE AND SUICIDAL BEHAVIOUR

Caring for aggressive patients, and those who wish to harm themselves, is always a matter of concern for nurses and doctors. Very often they are afraid of what may happen, particularly if a patient is violent or suicidal. In addition, behaviour of this kind always makes other patients in the ward feel anxious and insecure. The reaction of patients and staff to disturbed behaviour in the ward is quite understandable, particularly among nurses and doctors who have little experience of dealing with the problem. Aggressive and suicidal behaviour are not frequent occurrences in a psychiatric hospital, but the nurse should be aware of the difficulties involved, and the ways of preventing or dealing with them.

THE AGGRESSIVE PATIENT

Aggression is a normal response to certain situations, particularly when a person feels threatened and very afraid. Human beings appear naturally aggressive, as any teacher who has to deal with a class of six- or seven-year-olds will admit. A mature adult will have learned to control his natural aggression so that he can live more or less peaceably with other people. This does not mean that he will not lose his temper at times. There are many situations in which even the most well-controlled person will become angry, or even violent. If we think of the situations in which we could become angry, then we can discover those in which the mentally ill person can become hostile too.

THE CAUSES OF AGGRESSION

The causes of aggressive or violent behaviour in a person who is mentally ill are:

Brain damage. If certain areas of the brain are damaged by injury or disease, a patient may be prone to sudden aggressive outbursts, without apparent reason. Often, he will not realise what he is doing, and may not be able to remember afterwards. Brain damage is not a common cause of aggressive behaviour, but may sometimes be seen in epileptic patients (see Epilepsy, Chapter 11).

Failure of learning in childhood. There are some people who have never learned to control their natural aggression. Like children, they react to problems with anger and violence. The psychopathic patient may become aggressive because of his failure to learn self-control (see Psychopathic Disorder, Chapter 9).

Frustration. If a person is unable to do what he wants, or is prevented from doing it by other people, he can react by becoming angry or violent. A mentally ill patient may feel that he is being kept in hospital without good reason, and may become hostile towards the nursing staff. A patient who is overactive may become angry because other people are too slow for him, or will not let him have his own way. If a nurse refuses a request which the patient considers reasonable, or he feels ignored and neglected, he may easily become hostile or violent.

Anxiety and fear. If a patient is very anxious or afraid he may react with anger or violence. A mentally ill person may think that he will never leave hospital, or be scared of the treatment he might be given. Some patients are deluded, and become afraid of their imagined persecutors, or feel that other people are looking at them and talking about them behind their backs. Others are hallucinated, and may see horrible figures about to attack them, and attempt to defend themselves.

PREVENTION OF AGGRESSION

In many cases, aggressive or violent incidents can be avoided. The nurse can help to prevent them in the following ways:

Treat the patient with respect, **kindness and consideration**. This is a simple rule which generally works. No patient is so mentally ill that he is unable to appreciate kindness. It is known that nurses who treat patients with little regard and affection are usually the ones who have most problems with aggressive behaviour.

Give the patient as much freedom as possible. Frustration can be reduced by allowing the patient to go out of the ward as soon as he is well enough. He should be allowed to take decisions for himself, and should not be subjected to unnecessary rules. The nurse should agree to a patient's requests whenever possible. If a request has to be turned down, she should always tell him the reason for the decision.

Avoid situations which threaten the patient. Warning a patient to control his behaviour seldom works, and often makes him even more angry. The nurse must never threaten him with the use of treatments, such as injections or electrical treatment, or tell him that he will go to another ward if he does not behave.

Provide the patient with outlets for his aggressive feelings. Regular ward meetings between patients and staff often help to reduce aggressive incidents. If patients are allowed to release their feelings verbally they are less likely to resort to violence. Games, work and regular trips outside hospital also provide outlets for aggressive feelings. Sometimes it may be wiser to allow a patient to break a few cups, or a window, if it avoids a physical attack on someone else.

Ensure that the patient takes the medication prescribed for him. Tranquillizing drugs and sedatives help to calm the patient and make violence less likely.

Follow the advice given by the hospital authorities. The combined efforts of every member of the hospital team are essential if aggression is to be prevented. Many hospitals have special committees set up to deal with the problems of aggression, and to give advice about dealing with aggressive behaviour.

DEALING WITH VIOLENT BEHAVIOUR

If violent behaviour does occur in hospital, it may be necessary to restrain the patient. Physical restraint is only used for the following reasons:

1 To prevent the patient from harming himself or other people.

2   To separate the patient from others, or to remove dangerous
    articles from him.
3   To hold the patient while an injection is given, or to take him
    to a side room.

It is impossible to give the nurse exact guidance in dealing with
a violent patient, as every situation is different. She should be
guided by the particular rules of the hospital and the advice
issued by the Department of Health and Social Security, but
some general points are:

1   Never attempt to restrain a patient alone. There is always a
    risk that the nurse, or the patient, will be injured in this way.
2   Always summon help by calling, or if necessary leave the area
    to find help.
3   Each member of staff should try to take hold of one limb,
    holding them at the large joints. This is the best way to
    restrict the patient's movement without hurting him.
4   Maintain enough pressure to hold the patient still while an
    injection is given, or until he has calmed down.
5   If it is convenient, the patient can be wrapped in a blanket to
    control his movements, as this helps to prevent injury.

Every psychiatric hospital has rules to ensure that a disturbed
patient is not kept in a side room alone for long periods. In most
hospitals the doctor must give permission for a patient to be
secluded. The nurse should ensure that these rules are strictly
observed. After a violent incident it is important to discover if the
patient has sustained any injury. If he has, a doctor must be called
to examine him and prescribe treatment. A written report must
be made of all violent incidents and any injuries resulting from
them.

After the patient has calmed down he should always be given
an opportunity to talk about the incident. It is very important
that he should not feel that others are angry, or hold a grudge
against him. It is helpful if the ward team can meet to discuss an
aggressive incident soon after it occurs. Discussion may reveal the
cause of the problem and thus help to prevent further aggressive
behaviour.

THE SUICIDAL PATIENT

The nurse has the responsibility to protect a patient from self injury as far as possible. To do so, she must be aware of the risk of suicide in particular patients, and must know of the methods used to reduce this risk. Fortunately, suicide is not common, even in a psychiatric hospital. Some patients do, however, attempt suicide, and the methods they use vary. If a patient attempts to commit suicide in the hospital, it is usually by taking stored tablets, hanging or cutting blood vessels.

ASSESSING THE RISK OF SUICIDE

Most patients who are admitted to a psychiatric hospital have no intention of harming themselves. It is important that the nurse should be able to recognise those who may try to injure themselves deliberately, or attempt suicide. Suicide is more common among patients who are suffering from endogenous depression (see p. 77) or the early stages of Huntington's chorea (see p. 102). However, this does not mean that the nurse should ignore the possibility of suicide in patients suffering from other disorders.

A good impression of a patient's state of mind can generally be obtained by talking with him, listening to what he says, and careful observation. In her dealings with the patient the nurse should remember that he is more likely to be thinking of suicide under the following circumstances:

1 If he is very depressed and agitated (wringing his hands and pacing up and down the ward).
2 If he is deluded, particularly if he believes that he is dead or is suffering from a dreadful disease.
3 If he talks about suicide or his own death.
4 If he is unable to talk about his plans for the future or the things he may like to do.
5 If he often wakes in the early hours of the morning and cannot get back to sleep.
6 If he has tried to harm himself before.
7 If a relative or close friend has committed suicide.

8 If he suffers from a severe headache which has lasted for days or even weeks.

Any of the above points may indicate that the patient is a suicidal risk. If the nurse becomes aware of them she must report the matter immediately to the ward sister or doctor.

SUICIDAL GESTURES

Many people who attempt suicide do not really want to kill themselves. Some make a suicidal gesture as a desperate plea for help, or an attempt to alter their personal circumstances. Broken love affairs, financial losses and court appearances are some of the most common problems which may lead to a suicidal gesture. Frequently the attempt at suicide is planned so that the risk of death is small. Overdoses of drugs may be calculated, and the person may take them knowing that he will be discovered before it is too late. Those who frequently make suicidal gestures sometimes kill themselves by accident, or finally make a genuine attempt to end their lives. For this reason, all suicide attempts, or threats of suicide, must be taken seriously.

PRECAUTIONS

There are two methods of guarding against the possibility of a patient committing suicide in hospital. Which method is used depends upon the extent to which the patient is at risk. For this reason it is essential that the ward team should agree on the degree of risk and the care the patient will receive.

Constant observation or 'special care'
This method of care is used when the risk of a patient committing suicide is very great. The patient is put to bed in a side room, and a nurse must remain with him constantly. All dangerous articles, such as combs, scissors and razors are taken from him, and he must not be allowed to wear clothes with belts or cords. No glass, china, knives or other dangerous objects must be taken into his room. His meals should be served on plastic plates, and eaten

with a spoon. All his medication should be given in liquid form or by injection to ensure that he does not hide his drugs. All toilet facilities must be brought to him, and the patient must not be allowed to leave his room for any reason.

Constant observation is very stressful for the patient and the nurse. The patient will know that he is being guarded and may resent it. It is helpful if the nurse is able to talk with the patient and gain his confidence. He should be provided with books to read or some task which will help to keep him occupied. One nurse should not be allowed to remain with the patient for more than an hour at a time because of the danger that her attention will wander. The patient must be observed constantly until the doctor considers that the danger of suicide is less great.

Continuous observation
This method is used when the risk of suicide is not great enough to justify restricting the patient completely. All dangerous possessions must be taken from him, and he should be told not to leave the ward. It is often best to ask the patient to remain dressed in pyjamas and a dressing gown. The nurse should remain with him as much as possible, or be in the immediate vicinity. Talking with the patient, watching television with him, or joining him in occupational therapy will help him to feel that he is not being constantly watched. Even so it is impossible to observe a patient continuously without his knowledge. If the nurse explains that she is there because of the possibility that he might harm himself, the patient will generally accept it without ill feeling.

Unless the patient is restricted and constantly observed, there is always a risk that he will harm himself without being seen. Despite this, continuous observation is the most frequently used method of preventing suicide, and is generally successful. With the help of modern treatment for mental illness, both methods of observation seldom have to continue for long periods of time.

QUESTIONS

1 Give two possible causes of aggressive behaviour in a psychiatric patient.

2 Mention two ways in which a nurse can help to prevent aggression in a psychiatric hospital ward.

3 Give three reasons why an aggressive patient may need to be restrained.

4 Mention three observations which may lead you to believe that a patient is suicidal.

5 State two reasons why a patient may make a suicidal gesture.

6 Mention four precautions you would take when nursing a suicidal patient.

Chapter 15

INSTITUTIONALISM

It is well known that our immediate surroundings have a very great effect on our mood, attitudes and behaviour. It is more pleasant to be in a room which is well decorated and evenly lit than in one which is badly painted and dreary. The longer we have to spend in a particular place the more important it becomes to make it look bright, interesting and cheerful. Even so, no matter how pleasant our surroundings, sooner or later we feel the need for a change. For most people this need is met by taking holidays away from their usual environment.

The effect of living in the same dismal environment for years, with no opportunity for change, can be soul-destroying. This effect is known as institutionalism. It occurs most often in people who spend long periods in mental hospitals and prisons, but can also be seen in other institutions. It may sometimes occur in old-age pensioners and housewives who spend a long time at home with little opportunity to go out.

THE FEATURES OF INSTITUTIONALISM IN HOSPITAL PATIENTS

Institutionalism is usually a slow process, although some patients may become institutionalised in a matter of months. Institutionalised patients are often seen in the long-stay wards of psychiatric hospitals, where they become **dependent on the hospital** for their security and everyday needs.

The effects of institutionalism may vary. Some patients become mute and do nothing except sit in a chair all day. Others remain talkative and work hard, possibly in the ward kitchen or a hospital department. One of the earliest signs of institutionalism is a **loss of interest in the future**. If the patient is asked what he is going to do when he leaves hospital he may shrug his shoulders, make excuses or even argue against leaving. He has accepted that the future will be no different from the present, and little different from the past. Some patients become very withdrawn, particularly if they are not given any definite job to do. They lose interest in other patients because they in turn have lost interest. They find little point in speaking to people who do not care to answer.

An institutionalised patient is often very **submissive to the hospital staff**. He will do what is asked, however unfair, without complaining. He has accepted that it is pointless to argue if, in the end, you never win. Besides, it may be a good idea to please the staff as much as possible.

A lack of emotion may be obvious in the institutionalised patient. He has forgotten how to laugh, and does not cry. His answers are given automatically and without feeling. It is difficult for him to show enthusiasm for the same routine, the same faces, the same surroundings, year after year.

It is often said that a psychiatric patient can be recognised by his general appearance. This is not true, but an institutionalised patient often can be. **Neglect of personal appearance** is very common. The patient may not wash or shave properly, and will not bother to clean his shoes and change his clothes. He may walk with shuffling steps and with drooping head and shoulders. This **faulty posture** is doubtless a result of sitting too long in chairs with nothing to do, but gives the impression that the patient is a 'robot'.

THE CAUSES OF INSTITUTIONALISM

The causes of institutionalism in a psychiatric hospital are very complex. There are so many aspects of life in an institution that it is impossible to say which of them are responsible. All the factors mentioned here combine to cause institutionalism, but they can be grouped under three broad headings.

Isolation from the world outside hospital, and from relatives, friends and social events plays a great part in causing institutionalism. For most people life is made interesting and enjoyable by their relationships with others. Friends, relatives and colleagues help to keep a person mentally alert and interested in the future. A patient who is in a psychiatric hospital for a long time can seldom keep all his contacts with the world outside. He will probably have lost his job, and will certainly find it difficult to get another. The hospital may be a long distance from home, and after a time relatives may become tired of visiting him. Social events that the patient once looked forward to, such as birthdays, holidays, visits to the cinema or the local pub quickly vanish, and life becomes uninteresting. Although entertainments are provided in the hospital, they do not make up for the personal events which he has lost.

The longer the patient remains in hospital the greater is the chance that he will stay for good. If he cannot find a job it may be impossible to find somewhere to live. His relatives may not want him back home after a long time away, and landladies are often unwilling to let accommodation to a mental patient. Even if he finds a job, he may be very afraid of living in a room by himself with no friends. He may see life in hospital, no matter how hopeless, as being better than a life of loneliness in a bed-sitter.

The discipline and atmosphere of life in hospital can have a very great effect on the mood and behaviour of the patient. Large organisations can be very impersonal, and a patient can become one of a number very quickly. If the hospital is over-crowded, less attention can be given to individual patients. Some hospital buildings are old fashioned and depressing and make it obvious to patients that they are in an institution.

Long-stay patients may have their clothing provided by the hospital. If all the materials are similar, or the clothes are marked with the name of the hospital, patients are constantly reminded that their clothes are not their own. Personal clothing is important if pride and independence are to be maintained.

The feeling of hopelessness, which is a part of institutionalism, is a vicious circle. If doctors and nurses feel that little can be done for their patients, the patients become more apathetic and there is no improvement. If the patients do not improve, medical and nursing staff may feel that the situation is hopeless.

Certain restrictions are necessary in any organisation. A hospital could not function without discipline, but unnecessary discipline can be harmful to patients. Taking away a newly admitted patient's clothes and giving him a bath not because it is necessary, but because it is the rule, is one example of unnecessary discipline.

Nursing and medical staff often take decisions for the long-stay patient, leaving him little choice. The decisions are always taken with the patient's best interest in view, often because he is considered to be too ill to understand what he wants. There are, in fact, very few patients who are so mentally ill that they cannot make even simple decisions for themselves. If all decisions are taken away from a patient it will not be long before he is unable to think for himself.

A boring routine, month after month, will make patients dependent and apathetic. Many patients in long-stay wards sit in chairs for much of the day, with nothing to do, and spend long hours in bed. It is often difficult to find enough work on the ward to occupy every patient, particularly if a routine is established.

Meal times, which for most people form a high spot in the day, soon become routine to long-stay patients. Meals are usually prepared in a large kitchen, and easily become uninteresting, particularly if there is no choice.

In many long-stay wards it is difficult for patients to wash in private. If well designed bathing facilities are not available, all patients may have to take a bath at a fixed time during the week. This can be upsetting at first to people who were used to comfortable surroundings at home.

Patients who take no exercise and do little work during the day often find it difficult to sleep at night. They may be prescribed sedative drugs, but these can lead to further tiredness and disinterest during the day.

PREVENTION OF INSTITUTIONALISM

Prevention is better than cure. Institutionalism is extremely difficult to treat, and it is much better to prevent it happening in the first place. It is a mistake to believe that institutionalism only occurs in patients in long-stay wards, for sometimes the process begins shortly after admission. If it is to be avoided, the hospital team must be aware of the problem, and every member of staff must join in the effort to deal with it. Many large hospitals are now aware of the problem of institutionalism and have taken steps to avoid it. Reduction of overcrowding, improvement of buildings and an active occupational programme for patients are essential if institutionalism is not to be produced. The nurse can make a valuable contribution to the effort in many ways, and she must always be aware that her actions have a very great effect upon her patients.

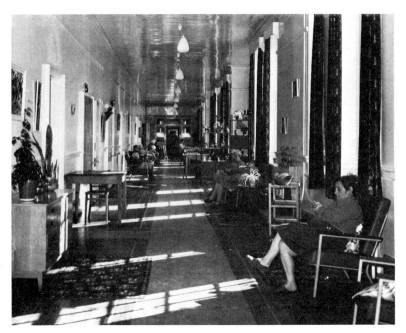

iv A long-stay ward in a psychiatric hospital

Much can be done to prevent the new patient from becoming isolated by encouraging his relatives and friends to visit him regularly. The longer the patient seems likely to remain in hospital the more important this is. Relatives and friends are more likely to visit if they receive a warm welcome from the nursing staff and are made to feel that their visits are necessary. The nurse should get to know visitors individually as this always encourages them to see the patient more frequently. The patient, too, will feel better if he sees that his visitors are able to get along well with the nursing staff. Visiting times should be as flexible as possible so that visitors are not put off by awkward hours. Old-age pensioners and other visitors with a limited income can often be helped to pay their fares to the hospital by the Department of Health and Social Security. Visitors receiving Supplementary Benefit can have the cost of their fares refunded by the hospital authorities. These facts should be mentioned to those people who find it difficult to visit regularly because of the cost of travelling long distances.

Regular visits home, sometimes for a few days, are important if the patient in hospital is to maintain contact with the world outside. The doctor will decide when the patient is well enough to go home for a short visit, and relatives should be told in advance. Patients who are unable to go home, or have no home to go to, should be encouraged to join other patients for outings as soon as they are well enough.

The first impression the new patient gains of the hospital is largely determined by the nursing staff. The way he is treated at first has a great bearing on his future progress. He should be greeted in a friendly, cheerful way, and the admission procedure should be as informal as possible. If his possessions must be checked, the nurse should explain why this has to be done. Routine searching of patients is seldom necessary unless they are very depressed, excited or confused. The patient should be allowed to keep as many of his personal possessions as possible. His clothes should not be locked away unless it is absolutely necessary. There is no need to give every patient a bath on admission to hospital. This can be very humiliating to some patients, especially if they are watched by a nurse. Only if a patient is very dirty or neglected should he be given a bath, and even then it does not have to be given a few minutes after admission. Doctors should not complain about having to examine the occasional dirty patient in a psychiatric admission ward.

The new patient should not be put to bed immediately unless it is absolutely essential. If possible, he should be given a choice of where he wants to sleep. Many people do not like certain foods, and the patient should be asked if there is anything he does not like eating. Even the largest hospital kitchen will arrange alternative meals on request.

Most admission wards provide a range of occupations and activities, and the new patient should be encouraged to join in these as soon as he is able. The domestic work can be shared by the patients on a weekly rota basis. Games such as table tennis and snooker should be available to keep patients occupied and active. Ward meetings for patients and staff are an essential part of treatment, and the new patient should be asked to attend these regularly. There he will get to know the other patients, and will be able to contribute to the running of the ward. Occupational therapy (see p. 191) is an important treatment, and the patient may be sent to a department of this kind in the hospital. The nurse should be aware of all the activities available for patients and encourage them to take part in as many as possible. Institutionalism can only be prevented with the aid of activity and interest on the part of patients and nurses.

QUESTIONS

1   What do you understand by the term 'institutionalism'?
2   What observations would lead you to believe that a patient was institutionalised?
3   List three causes of institutionalism in a psychiatric hospital.
4   What can you do to help prevent a newly admitted patient from becoming institutionalised?
5   Why should the nurse try to develop good relationships with patients' visitors?

Chapter 16

THE TREATMENT OF MENTAL ILLNESS

In an earlier chapter we have learned that there is seldom a single, definite cause of mental illness. We shall not be surprised to learn, therefore, that there is equally seldom a single, definite treatment.

In a general hospital, patients are usually given specific treatments for the illnesses they have. The doctor generally knows how the treatment works, and the patient co-operates with the doctor and nurses in order to get better. In a psychiatric hospital there are few treatments which work effectively every time. Indeed, most patients are given more than one treatment, and these treatments vary as much from patient to patient as from one sort of illness to another. We do not know exactly how many of the treatments for mental illness work; only that they do. Unlike the patients in a general hospital, some psychiatric patients do not want treatment and may not co-operate with the doctor and nurses. Some do not realise they are ill and may actively resist all forms of treatment.

The nurse has an extremely important role to play in the treatment of the mentally ill. She is always in much closer contact with the patient than any other member of the hospital team, and has a greater opportunity to get to know him and report on his improvement. Her actions, attitudes and the skills she develops to help him deal with his problems are themselves essential parts of his treatment.

The treatments for mental illness can be divided into two main groups, psychological treatments and physical treatments. Whatever mental illness they have, most patients will be treated with one or more from both groups.

PSYCHOLOGICAL TREATMENT

PSYCHOTHERAPY

When we talk with a friend about a particular problem he may have, we are almost certainly, without knowing it, practising the art of psychotherapy. We listen to what our friend says, and talk with him in an understanding and reassuring way. Psychotherapy, when used as a treatment for mental illness, is more specialised than this, but basically it is treatment by **listening** to what the patient says and **talking** with him.

Psychotherapy is used individually with the patient and doctor talking alone, or in groups comprised of patients, nurses and doctors.

Individual psychotherapy helps the patient by encouraging him to discover for himself the reasons for his behaviour. The doctor listens to the patient and offers explanation and advice when necessary. By these means he helps the patient to come to a greater understanding of himself and to find a way of dealing with his problems. Individual psychotherapy sessions usually take place at regular intervals, and many patients are treated over a period of some weeks or months.

Group psychotherapy is just as effective as individual psychotherapy, and it allows the doctor to see several patients at one time. The patients, generally between eight and twelve in number, learn from each other as well as the therapist.

The new patient who joins a group may feel too embarrassed to talk about his difficulties at first. After a time, he will begin to feel more at ease, and by listening to others come to see that his problems are not unique. Eventually, when he feels more confident in the group he will begin to talk about his problems, and will find that other patients are willing to listen and give him advice. The advantage of group psychotherapy is that it helps patients to develop relationships with each other. This is important because, at least to some degree, all mentally ill people experience difficulties in their relationships with others.

The group therapist is usually a psychiatrist, psychologist or specially trained psychiatric nurse. The part he takes in the group

depends very much on his own beliefs and personality. He may
say very little, allowing the patients to do most of the talking, or he
may spend much of the time explaining behaviour and offering
advice. The role of the nurse in group therapy depends largely
on the wishes of the therapist. In some groups nurses are
encouraged to talk, while in others they are asked to listen and
only respond to direct questions from a patient.

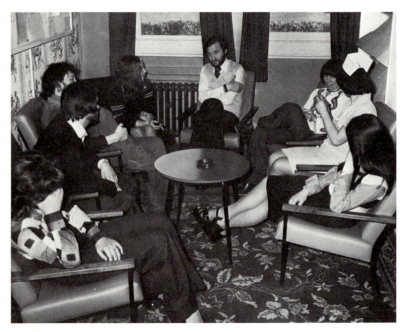

v Group psychotherapy in progress

To some extent every psychiatric nurse uses psychotherapy in
her dealings with patients. Almost every mentally ill person will
need to talk about himself and his problems, and it is the nurse's
job to listen and give him support and encouragement. Although
she is not a trained psychotherapist, the ward nurse must be aware
that the way she relates to him is of the greatest importance. The
skill of listening and talking with patients in a meaningful way
can only be learned by experience and by willingness to understand human problems and feelings.

PSYCHOANALYSIS

Psychoanalysis was introduced by Sigmund Freud, and is a very formal and intense method of psychotherapy. The patient sees the analyst regularly, usually several times a week over a period of months or years. During the interview, the patient lies on a couch and is encouraged to say whatever comes into his mind. This technique is called **free association**. The analyst will also ask the patient to recall his recent dreams, and will help him to understand their meaning. By these methods the analyst is able to help the patient uncover many of the unconscious memories which may be responsible for his illness. Psychoanalysis is a very expensive and time consuming form of treatment. It is not widely used in psychiatric hospitals in the United Kingdom.

Very often the patient who is receiving psychoanalysis or psychotherapy develops feelings towards the therapist which are similar to those he once had for his parents, brothers and sisters. This situation is known as **transference**. The patient behaves towards the therapist as he once did towards people who were important to him as a child. He may treat the therapist with deep regard and affection or with anger and jealousy. The transference situation is used by the therapist to help the patient understand his difficulties and feelings.

Transference also occurs in the nurse–patient relationship. Very often a patient will unconsciously associate the nurse with his mother or father, and behave towards her accordingly. This helps to explain why a patient may come to like or dislike a particular nurse for no apparent reason.

HYPNOSIS

Hypnosis was made popular by the German physician, Friedrich Mesmer, (1733–1815) who used to give public displays of his magical powers in Paris. By putting his subjects into a trance, he was able to make them behave as he commanded, and supposedly cure their illnesses. Although Mesmer was declared a fraud and ceased to practise his 'cures', hypnotism is still sometimes used to treat neurotic illnesses.

By talking softly to the patient, and sometimes by asking him to gaze at an object in front of him such as a pencil, the hypnotist is able to put him into a trance, or artificial sleep. The patient can then be encouraged to talk about repressed experiences, or the hypnotist can put suggestions into his mind.

BEHAVIOUR THERAPY

Behaviour therapy is a psychological treatment used to relieve the patient's symptoms rather than deal with their cause. It is based on the theory that unwanted patterns of behaviour can be removed by associating them with something unpleasant, and that new behaviour can be learned if it is associated with pleasant feelings.

When training a dog, its owner praises it when it obeys and smacks it when it disobeys. The dog learns that some actions bring reward and others bring pain. This learning is known as **conditioning**. In the treatment of mental illness conditioning is used in a highly specialised form.

A type of behaviour therapy called **desensitisation** is often used to treat phobic anxiety (see p. 60). The patient is interviewed by the therapist, and together they make a list of all the situations in which the patient becomes anxious. The list is then graded according to the degree of anxiety produced by each situation. For example, a patient who is afraid of cats may feel panic stricken at the thought of a cat jumping on his lap, but only slightly worried about seeing a cat in the street. In this case 'cat jumping on lap' would be at the top of the list, and 'seeing cat in the street' would appear somewhere near the end.

At subsequent interviews the therapist teaches the patient to relax, and asks him to imagine the situation which produces least anxiety. Gradually he works through the list until the patient can imagine himself in the most terrifying of them without anxiety. Having learned a new pattern of behaviour in imagination, the patient must then carry what he has learned into everyday life.

Aversion therapy is another form of behaviour therapy which attempts to alter unwanted behaviour by associating it with unpleasant experiences. It is most often used in the treatment of alcoholism (see p. 125).

The alcoholic patient is given a drug which will make him sick (an emetic drug) such as apomorphine, or a drug which will make him feel ill if he drinks alcohol, e.g. disulfiram (Antabuse). He is then given his favourite drink until he begins to vomit and feels physically ill. No attempt is made to wash the patient, and he is deliberately allowed to feel wretched. A check on his pulse rate and blood pressure should be made at intervals because of the danger of collapse, and the equipment for the care of an unconscious patient must be available during treatment.

Some doctors prefer to use electric shocks or other painful stimuli in aversion therapy. If the patient continues to associate the unpleasant feelings with alcohol, he will give up drink. Unlike desensitisation, which is highly successful, the results of aversion therapy are often very poor. This is because it is more difficult to persuade a person to give up something he likes doing than to teach him to do something he wants to do. Many doctors consider that aversion therapy is barbaric, and refuse to undertake this treatment.

Token economy is a type of behaviour therapy sometimes used to improve the behaviour and appearance of long-stay, institutionalised patients. Usually every patient in the ward is involved, and supplied with token money which can be used to buy food, drink and cigarettes from the hospital shop. Whenever a patient shows a sign of improvement, such as washing himself, polishing his shoes or attempting conversation, the nurse rewards him by giving him extra tokens. The patient learns that the more he does for himself the richer he becomes, and the more he can buy and enjoy.

Nurses and doctors often claim that token economy is very successful, and report great improvements in their patients. There is, however, the danger that the very rigid system does little to rehabilitate long-stay patients, but simply substitutes one form of institutional behaviour for another. The system does benefit very deteriorated patients who may later be able to take part in more active rehabilitation programmes (see Institutionalism, Chapter 15, and Rehabilitation, Chapter 17).

PHYSICAL TREATMENTS

TREATMENT WITH DRUGS (CHEMOTHERAPY)

The use of drugs in the treatment of mental illness dates from the earliest times. Until the beginning of this century few of these drugs were of any real benefit, and some were positively harmful. Great advances have been made during the last seventy years, and today there are drugs which are extremely effective in the treatment of mental disorder. These modern drugs can be divided into three large groups; sedatives and hypnotics, tranquillizers, and antidepressants.

Sedatives and hypnotics are drugs which have a calming effect and help patients to sleep. There is really no difference between a drug which is a sedative, and one which is a hypnotic. If the drug is given during the day to calm the patient it is called a sedative, and if a higher dose is given at night to help him sleep it is called a hypnotic. These drugs are useful to patients who are extremely anxious, agitated and find it difficult to sleep.

Many sedative and hypnotic drugs contain barbiturate. These barbiturate drugs may be short acting, medium acting or long acting. A patient who finds it difficult to get off to sleep may benefit from a short acting barbiturate which works quickly. Someone who gets off to sleep easily but who wakes up in the early hours will benefit from a long acting barbiturate which takes effect some hours after he has swallowed it. Examples of the different types of barbiturate drugs are quinalbarbitone sodium (Seconal) 50–100 mg (short acting), amylobarbitone sodium (Sodium Amytal) 200–400 mg (medium acting) and barbitone sodium (Medinal) 300–600 mg (long acting).

Barbiturate drugs sometimes produce undesirable results called **side effects**. One of these is a severe 'hangover' in the morning, which makes the drugs unsuitable for elderly, confused patients. Barbiturates should always be used carefully for patients suffering from heart or respiratory disease, as they can sometimes depress respiration. Certain other drugs, including alcohol, can make the effect of barbiturates more powerful, and the combination can be dangerous. Used over a long period of time, barbiturate drugs can lead to addiction (see pp. 119 and 122). Large supplies of the drug should never be given to patients for use at home, as overdosage of barbiturates is one of the most common methods of suicide.

Many doctors prefer to prescribe the safer and less addictive non-barbiturate drugs. Their side effects are less severe, making them safer for elderly patients. Non-barbiturate sedatives and hypnotics include nitrazepam (Mogadon) 5–10 mg, dichloralphenazone (Welldorm) 650–1,300 mg, triclofos (Tricloryl) 1,000–2,000 mg and chloral hydrate (Noctec) 500–1,000 mg.

The tranquillizers are a large group of drugs which make the patient feel less anxious without putting him to sleep, and which help to abolish hallucinations and delusions. The drugs can be divided into two basic types, the **major tranquillizers** and the **minor tranquillizers**.

The *major tranquillizers* are used to treat psychotic patients and those who are extremely anxious or agitated. Most of them belong to the group of chemical compounds known as **phenothiazines**. Some examples of phenothiazines are chlorpromazine (Largactil) 50–500 mg, thioridazine (Melleril) 50–500 mg, trifluoperazine (Stelazine) 2–30 mg, perphenazine (Fentazin) 4–24 mg and promazine (Sparine) 25–300 mg daily. All of these drugs can be given in tablet and syrup form, and most of them can be given by intra-muscular injection if required.

Phenothiazines are often given to patients in very high doses, and all of them, particularly chlorpromazine, can produce side effects. The common side effects of major tranquillizers include:

drowsiness
Parkinsonian symptoms (tremor, stiffness of the limbs, short, quick steps when walking)
dermatitis
photosensitivity (sensitivity to sunlight) resulting in a skin rash or burns
jaundice
obesity

postural hypotension (a fall in blood pressure when the patient
stands up)
urinary retention

If a patient who is taking a phenothiazine drug appears
jaundiced or complains of a sort throat, no further drugs should
be given, and a doctor must be informed immediately. Similar
action should be taken if the patient appears unusually drowsy, or
complains of dizziness or difficulty in passing urine. Burns can
often be prevented by asking the patient to avoid strong sunlight,
or by providing him with a sun deflectant cream which can be
applied to exposed parts of the body. The Parkinsonian symptoms can be reduced if the patient is prescribed a **rigidity** and
tremor controller such as procyclidine (Kemadrin) 2·5–30 mg,
benzhexol (Artane) 1–15 mg or orphenadrine (Disipal) 50–400 mg
daily. The nurse must be aware that she too can develop a severe
skin rash by handling phenothiazine drugs. This can be avoided
by wearing gloves, particularly when preparing injections or
pouring syrup.

Long acting phenothiazines are sometimes given to patients
who are discharged from hospital but still need medication, and
to those who cannot be relied upon to take tablets. The drugs
are given by intramuscular injection, and are effective for two to
six weeks. The dose and frequency of the injection is adjusted by
the doctor to suit individual patients. The long acting phenothiazine drugs are fluphenazine decanoate (Modecate), fluphenazine enanthate (Moditen) and flupenthixol decanoate (Depixol).

A major tranquillizing drug which is not a phenothiazine is
haloperidol (Serenace). It is given in doses of 1·5–20 mg daily, and
is useful in the treatment of schizophrenia and hypomania. The
side effects of haloperidol are similar to those of the phenothiazine
drugs.

The *minor tranquillizers* are used in the treatment of anxiety
states and other neurotic illnesses. They are not phenothiazines,
and severe side effects seldom occur. Some examples of minor
tranquillizers are diazepam (Valium) 6–60 mg, lorazepam
(Ativan) 1–10 mg and chlordiazepoxide (Librium) 10–30 mg
daily.

The antidepressants, as the name suggests, help to combat depression. They are frequently used in the treatment of all types of depressive illness, and are considered to be very effective drugs.

Antidepressants can be divided into two groups. The first group, called **tricyclic** antidepressants, are chemically related to the phenothiazines. Some examples of tricyclic drugs are imipramine (Tofranil) 50–150 mg, amitriptyline (Tryptizol) 50–300 mg, doxepin (Sinequan) 30–300 mg and clomipramine (Anafranil) 50–200 mg daily.

The second group of antidepressants, called Monoamine Oxidase Inhibitors (M.A.O.I.s), have a definite effect on the chemistry of the brain. Examples of these drugs are nialamide (Niamid) 75–150 mg and phenelzine (Nardil) 30–60 mg daily. Because of the danger of severe hypertension, patients who are prescribed M.A.O.I.s must not take certain drugs and foods. The foods which they must not eat are Bovril, Marmite, Oxo, cheese, broad beans, yoghurt and pickled herrings. All alcoholic drink must also be avoided. To avoid the risk that other drugs may be given to the patient in an emergency, he is required to carry a card with him which states that he is taking M.A.O.I.s. He must be instructed to show the card to any doctor or dentist before he accepts treatment.

ANAFRANIL INFUSION THERAPY

The antidepressant drug, clomipramine (Anafranil) may be given by intravenous infusion. A course of treatment, called Anafranil Infusion Therapy, is useful to selected patients who suffer from obsessive-compulsive neurosis, phobic anxiety or reactive depression (see Chapter 6).

The infusion is given on five days a week, and a course of treatment may last for two or three weeks. Usually the patient is given 50 mg of Anafranil on the first day, and the dose is then increased daily to a maximum of 250–350 mg. The maximum dose is reached half-way through the course, after which the amount is reduced each day. The last infusion contains only 50 mg of the drug. The course of treatment is generally given to in-patients, although most are encouraged to return home at week-ends. Those returning home during treatment are required to take tablets of Anafranil while away from hospital.

For the daily treatment, the necessary equipment for an intravenous infusion is prepared. The required dose of Anafranil is introduced with a sterile syringe into 300–500 ml of normal saline infusion fluid. The container should be shaken slightly to ensure that the drug is well mixed. The patient is made comfortable on a bed, and covered with a blanket. The nurse checks and

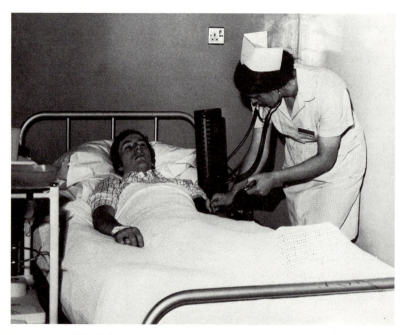

VI Anafranil infusion therapy. The nurse must monitor the infusion and record the patient's pulse and blood pressure every thirty minutes

records the patient's pulse and blood pressure, and if these are within normal limits the doctor inserts a cannula into a vein in his forearm. Having excluded air from the giving set, the cannula is connected, and the infusion is given at a rate of approximately forty-five drips a minute. During treatment the nurse must monitor the rate of the drip, and check and record the patient's pulse and blood pressure every thirty minutes. If the drip is interrupted, or the patient appears unwell, the nurse must stop the infusion and inform the doctor immediately.

Anafranil Infusion Therapy is usually not unpleasant, although a new patient may require reassurance at first. Many patients feel relaxed after a time and are willing to talk about their problems during treatment. Others feel drowsy much of the time and may go to sleep while the infusion is in progress. Before beginning a course of treatment, the doctor will tell the patient that he may experience some side effects of the drug. These are a dry mouth, tremor, nausea and occasionally vomiting. The side effects can be reduced by giving the patient diazepam (Valium) 5 mg three times daily.

Anafranil Infusion Therapy is usually given to four or five patients at one time. This small number ensures that treatment is given in a relaxed atmosphere, and that the patient has every opportunity to talk to the nurse or doctor if he wishes. Some hospitals have a special clinic which is used only for this form of treatment.

ABREACTION

Abreaction means a release of pent-up emotion. As a form of treatment in hospital abreaction is produced by drugs or gases, and is useful for patients who are too shy or anxious to express their emotions normally.

It is well known that a person who is normally shy may express what he really feels after having too much to drink. Alcohol is not used for this purpose in hospital, but intravenous injections of barbiturate drugs, or inhalations of ether or carbon dioxide and oxygen have a similar effect. As well as being a method of treatment, abreaction can be used to diagnose mental illness, particularly when a patient is not willing to talk freely.

ELECTRO-CONVULSIVE THERAPY (E.C.T.)

Electro-convulsive Therapy (often referred to as E.C.T., Electroplexy or simply Electrical Treatment) is a way of producing a fit, similar to an epileptic fit, by passing electricity through the patient's brain. It is a widely used and effective treatment for depression, and occasionally for some other mental illnesses. The patient is given a general anaesthetic before treatment and feels no pain. E.C.T. is normally very safe, the only complication being slight memory loss and confusion for a time after treatment.

When a doctor decides to recommend E.C.T., he will first of all discuss the treatment with the patient and his relatives. He will explain that a course of treatment usually lasts for three to six weeks, and is generally given twice a week. As most patients find the thought of having electricity passed through the head distressing, the doctor must always be prepared to answer questions tactfully and truthfully. When he has the agreement of the patient and his relations, he will ask them to sign a consent form for the administration of the general anaesthetic. He will then give the patient a thorough medical examination, and arrange for a chest X-ray, blood and urine tests if these have not already been done.

Most hospitals have an E.C.T. clinic, and treatment is usually given in the morning. The patient is not allowed anything to eat or drink for eight hours before treatment, although some doctors will allow one cup of tea at breakfast time. Routine medication is not usually given on the morning of treatment. A nurse should accompany the patient to the clinic, and remain with him in the waiting room. She should talk to the patient, perhaps about the morning news or a magazine article, to help relieve his anxiety. Before entering the treatment room he should be asked to empty his bladder. In some hospitals a subcutaneous injection of atropine (0·5–1 mg) is given before treatment to dry up secretions in the respiratory tract, relax bronchial muscles and increase the heart rate.

In the treatment room the patient is asked to remove dentures, glasses, hairclips and sharp jewellery. All tight clothing is loosened, and he lies on the bed in the supine position, his head supported by one small pillow. The anaesthetist injects a solution of the anaesthetic (e.g. methohexitone sodium (Brietal) 50–120 mg) into a vein in the patient's forearm. As soon as he is asleep, a muscle relaxant (e.g. suxamethonium chloride (Scoline) 20–100 mg) is injected through the same needle. The muscle relaxant paralyses the patient's muscles so that he will not have a severe convulsion, and thus reduces the risk of fractures. The drug also paralyses the respiratory muscles, and so is given after the anaesthetic to ensure that the patient does not have the experience of being unable to breathe.

As soon as the patient is fully asleep the anaesthetist inflates his lungs with oxygen and inserts a mouth gag. The E.C.T. machine is brought to the bedside, and the electrodes, which are

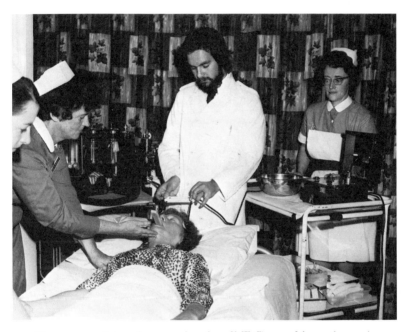

VII Electo-convulsive therapy showing E.T.C. machine, electrodes and oxygen apparatus

attached to a headset and soaked in an electrolyte solution, are applied to the patient's temples. The doctor or nurse presses a button on the headset which allows the current to pass through, and the fit takes place immediately. Because the patient's muscles are paralysed all that can be noticed is a slight twitching of his face, fingers and toes. The electric current which passes through

his brain is not very powerful. It is just strong enough to light a
100 watt, 240 volt electric light bulb for a moment or two.

The electrodes are removed from the patient's head, and when
the fit has stopped the mouth gag is taken out. The anaesthetist
ventilates his lungs with oxygen by using a re-breathing bag,
until he can breathe by himself. When the patient is breathing
normally he is placed on a trolley, with his head turned to one
side, and wheeled into the recovery room.

A nurse must be constantly in attendance until the patient is
fully recovered. The necessary equipment for the care of an unconscious patient should always be at hand. If there is any marked
change in the patient's colour, pulse or respiration, or the nurse
notices that he is sweating or thinks he is about to vomit, a doctor
must be summoned immediately. Usually the patient wakes up
quite quickly. When fully awake he should be given a cup of tea,
and afterwards helped into an armchair. When he is able to walk
steadily, the nurse should accompany him back to the ward.

The loss of memory which follows E.C.T. varies from one
patient to another. Some patients will be very confused for
several hours, while others will quickly recover from their loss of
memory. Most patients ask questions after treatment, such as
'Where am I?', 'What has happened?' or 'What day is it?' The
nurse must always answer the questions, even if they are repeated
again and again. The patient should be told that he has had
E.C.T., his belongings should be returned to him, and he should
be encouraged to talk with other patients he knows in the ward.
The nurse can mention familiar names and places to him as this
will help to prompt his memory. While the patient remains
confused, a nurse must stay with him to ensure that he does not
wander away from the ward or injure himself.

In an attempt to reduce memory loss after E.C.T., some
doctors prefer to place the electrodes on one side of the patient's
head during treatment. This method of producing a fit is called
unilateral E.C.T. The side of the head on which the electrodes
are placed depends on whether the patient is right- or left-handed.
If he is right-handed the electrodes are placed on the right side,
and if he is left-handed they are placed on the left. Although
unilateral E.C.T. does help to prevent confusion in many patients,

a longer course of treatment may be required before the mental condition improves.

QUESTIONS

1 What do you understand by the term 'psychotherapy'?
2 What is meant by the word 'transference'?
3 What do you understand by the term 'behaviour therapy'?
4 Name a mental illness which may be treated by desensitisation.
†5 Name the physical methods of treatment for mental disorders.
*6 Name two tranquillizing drugs.
*7 Name a drug which controls muscular tremor. Give an example of how it might be used for a psychiatric patient.
8 Name two antidepressant drugs and state their usual dosages.
9 What information should the nurse give to a patient who has been prescribed a Monoamine Oxidase Inhibitor (M.A.O.I.)?
10 Name a mental illness which may be relieved by electro-convulsive therapy.
*11 Name the drugs that may be used in the course of electro-convulsive therapy.
12 What complications can arise after electro-convulsive therapy?

* Reproduced by permission of The General Nursing Council for England and Wales.
† Reproduced by permission of The Northern Ireland Council for Nurses and Midwives.

Chapter 17

REHABILITATION

The aim of rehabilitation is to return the patient to a normal life outside hospital. He will have been admitted to hospital because, for one reason or another, he was no longer able to cope with life in society. The physical treatments such as drugs or E.C.T. will help to relieve his mental illness, and the specific psychological treatments and his relationships with the nursing staff will help him to deal more effectively with his problems. However, his improvement will only be maintained if he is given the necessary support and encouragement on the road back to the world outside hospital.

Rehabilitation involves training and educating the patient to deal more successfully with his problems, giving general support and guidance in times of difficulty, and sometimes altering his environment. Not every patient will require help in quite the same way. The neurotic patient may require help in planning how to use his leisure time, or with his personal relationships, while the long-stay schizophrenic may need encouragement to develop work habits and to care for his personal appearance. A rehabilitation programme must be designed to meet the needs of the individual patient. It is important to discover the areas in which he needs help, so that the programme can be planned accordingly.

In every psychiatric hospital there are departments which have the special function of helping patients to prepare for discharge from hospital. They are sometimes grouped together under the heading of the 'Rehabilitation Service', and usually a psychiatrist, a nurse administrator and an occupational therapist are appointed to plan and organise the work of the various departments. Patients who may benefit from rehabilitation are referred to one or other of the departments by a consultant psychiatrist.

OCCUPATIONAL THERAPY

The importance of keeping patients occupied in hospital has been mentioned earlier, but occupational therapy should be more than a method of preventing boredom. Everyone has a need for self-expression, and creative, interesting work can be a source of great pleasure to many patients. Very often a patient is able to learn a new skill during his stay in hospital and, perhaps for the first time for many years, feels the pride and satisfaction that comes from personal achievement. Patients working at occupational therapy usually do so in groups, and this provides opportunity for learning how best to get along with other people.

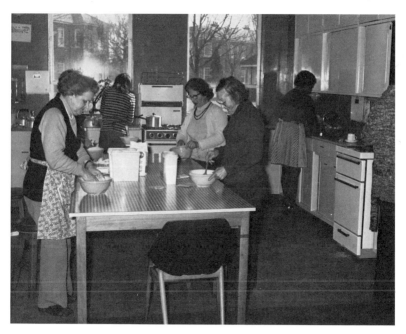

VIII A cookery session, one of many interesting and useful activities in the occupational therapy department

Occupational therapy provides many interesting and rewarding jobs for patients to do, of which painting, woodwork, needlework, typing and cooking are just a few. Leisure activities such as dancing, keep fit classes, discussion groups and music appreciation are also included in the occupational therapy programme, and these can help patients to plan better use of their leisure time.

Occupational therapy can be valuable in helping institutionalised patients to readjust to the world outside hospital. Many of these patients have forgotten how to cook, shop, handle money and care for their personal hygiene. Occupational therapy can help them to re-learn these skills and re-awaken interest in their surroundings and other people.

Occupational therapy is usually conducted in a special department within the hospital, and most hospitals have a staff of trained occupational therapists and helpers. Very often, members of the department come regularly to the wards to help those patients who are unable to go to the department itself. Nurses spend some time during their training working alongside occupational therapists, and the experience they gain can be of great value in helping them to care for their patients.

INDUSTRIAL THERAPY

Industrial therapy provides patients with tasks similar to those undertaken by many people who earn a living outside hospital. Most psychiatric hospitals have industrial therapy departments, which are usually organised in a similar way to a workshop or factory. In these departments patients are trained to complete jobs efficiently, and encouraged to develop work habits which will help them to gain employment outside. Usually they are paid a small wage which varies according to their performance.

Most hospitals are unable to provide work suitable for job training, and the aim of industrial therapy is to train patients to work efficiently rather than teach a particular skill. Nevertheless, industrial therapy can provide interesting work for patients, many jobs being supplied by large companies outside hospital. After satisfactory training, the patient who is ready to be discharged can be referred to a Government Training Centre to be taught a new skill or occupation.

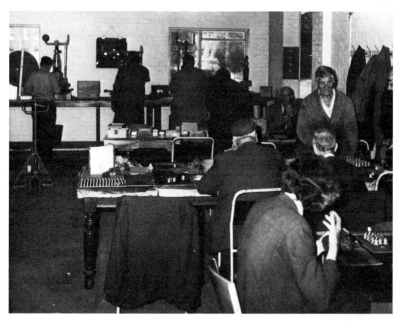

ix A workshop in the industrial therapy department. The patients are assembling machine parts for a local factory

RECREATIONAL THERAPY

Recreation is important for everyone, and not least for the patient in a psychiatric hospital. It provides interest and enjoyment, and a welcome change from daily routine. Many patients will have found it hard to enjoy social activities in the community, often because of difficulty in relating to other people. Social activities in hospital can help them to overcome their shyness and provide opportunities to develop personal relationships.

Recreational activities must be carefully chosen to suit the needs of the individual patient, and he should be given as much freedom of choice as possible. Elderly patients will often enjoy listening to old-time music, playing card games or bingo, or simply talking to each other during afternoon tea. Younger patients will enjoy modern dancing, socials, and sports such as cricket and football. Outings to places of interest, films, concerts and library facilities should be available to everyone.

In many hospitals a nursing officer is responsible for the organisation of all recreational activities. Occupational therapists and voluntary service organisers can also make a large contribution, and the involvement of nurses in this aspect of patient care is of the utmost importance.

CARE IN THE COMMUNITY

Rehabilitation does not necessarily end when the patient is discharged from hospital. The period immediately after leaving hospital can be very difficult for some patients, and a great deal of help may be required from the hospital and community services.

The two greatest problems for the patient about to leave hospital are those of finding work and accommodation. The Rehabilitation Officer may be able to help the patient find a job and somewhere to live before he leaves, or arrange for him to see other people in the community who are able to help. Some patients are of course able to return to their homes and employment, but even so the period of readjustment may be difficult. The help available to patients in the community can be grouped under three headings.

EMPLOYMENT

The local **Employment Service Agency** (**JobCentre**) keeps a list of available jobs in the area, and can arrange for an unemployed person to be interviewed for a suitable vacancy. The agency also has a **Disablement Resettlement Officer** (**D.R.O.**) who will help to find work for people who are mentally or physically disabled. If necessary, he will make an appointment for the patient to see him, or will arrange to visit him in hospital. The **Unemployment Benefit Office** pays an allowance to those people who cannot find suitable work.

Those patients who cannot return to their previous employment, if they are considered suitable, can be offered a place at a **Government Training Centre**. There they are taught a new skill or trade, and are paid an allowance during training.

Patients who are unable to work in the community can be referred to the local **Sheltered Workshop**. There they are given suitable work, and allowances are made for their particular difficulties.

ACCOMMODATION

The local authority, and some voluntary organisations, provide **hostels** for patients who cannot find their own accommodation. The hostels are usually supervised by trained staff who are able to give advice and help to patients when necessary.

Under the National Assistance Act of 1948, local authorities have to provide accommodation for patients with mental disorders. Because the law is contained in Part III of the Act, the homes are called **Part III Accommodation**. They are usually supervised by nurses or local authority workers. Unfortunately, the number of places available is not great enough to meet demands.

Hotels, owned by private individuals or companies, sometimes accept psychiatric patients as long-term residents. The service and facilities they provide vary widely.

Group homes, owned by the hospital authorities, league of friends or a housing association provide accommodation for long-stay patients. A small group of patients live together, pay rent for the house, and budget together for day-to-day expenses. The residents accept responsibility for their home with only the minimum of supervision.

SPECIALIST CARE

When a patient is discharged from hospital it is usually into the care of his **general practitioner** (Family Doctor). The G.P. will often know the patient and his family very well, and is therefore in a good position to advise him on any problems he may have. If the patient is taking medication regularly, the G.P. will usually issue the prescriptions. By seeing the patient regularly, the doctor is able to keep an accurate check on his progress.

Patients who are discharged from hospital are sometimes seen regularly by a psychiatrist at an **out-patient clinic**. The clinic is attached to the psychiatric hospital or the local general hospital. Out-patient appointments give the patient an opportunity to discuss problems with his psychiatrist, and enable the psychiatrist to adjust treatment if necessary.

Many psychiatric hospitals provide facilities for patients to attend hospital during the day, returning home at night. **Day hospitals** lend support to patients who are not ill enough to be admitted, and often provide some relief for relatives at home.

Social workers are specially trained people employed by the local authority. They are involved with the patient's family and background, and are able to provide the psychiatrist with important information. When the patient is discharged from hospital, the social worker may continue to visit him at home, and will try to assist with any social problem which may arise. Under the Mental Health Act, 1959, social workers are given special powers to sign applications for the hospital detention of the mentally ill.

Community psychiatric nurses are trained nurses who have special experience of caring for patients in the community. They are often based at the local psychiatric hospital, and visit patients in their homes regularly. During their visits they may administer drugs, make an assessment of the patient's condition, and give advice and help to the patient and his family. In an emergency they are able to call the doctor to prescribe or change medication, and if necessary they can bring the patient back to hospital to see a consultant.

Recent trends in the community care of the mentally ill have proved that with adequate facilities, many patients can be maintained outside hospital. There is no doubt that with early diagnosis, and the support of social workers and community nurses, large numbers of mentally ill people can be successfully treated without the need for admission to hospital.

QUESTIONS

1   What is the aim of rehabilitation?

2   What professional groups may be involved with rehabilitation in a psychiatric hospital?

3   List the advantages of occupational therapy.

*4 What are the duties of the Occupational Therapist?

5   List the advantages of industrial therapy.

*6 There are many activities which your hospital would describe as recreational therapy. Mention three of these.

7   State two recreational activities suitable for elderly patients.

8   Give two ways in which a day hospital can help in the care of the mentally ill.

*9 Mention two ways in which a social worker can help a newly discharged hospital patient.

10 What facilities exist to help a newly discharged patient find accommodation?

*11 After discharge, how may a patient be helped by the psychiatric out-patient department?

12 What are the functions of a community psychiatric nurse?

* Reproduced by permission of The General Nursing Council for England and Wales.

Index

Abreaction 185
Addiction to drugs, *see* drug dependence
Adolescence 23–5; problems of 24, 25
Adulthood 26–9
Adult training centre 147
Aggression: causes of 159, 160; prevention of 160, 161
Alcoholics Anonymous 128
Alcoholism 125–8; case illustration 128–32
Ambivalence 20
Amitriptyline 183
Amnesia: and E.C.T. 188; anterograde 46; hysterical 61; in senile dementia 99; retrograde 46
Amphetamine, misuse of 119
Amylobarbitone 180
Anafranil infusion therapy 183–5
Anorexia and mental illness 39
Anorexia nervosa 150, 151
Antabuse 127, 128, 179
Anticonvulsant therapy 138, 139
Antidepressants 183
Anxiety 42
Anxiety neurosis 57–9; case illustration 64–6
Apathy 42
Apomorphine 179
Arteriosclerotic dementia 103
Asthma 153
Atropine 186
Auditory hallucinations 45, 81
Automatism, post epileptic 134, 137
Aversion therapy 178, 179

Barbitone 180
Barbiturates 180, 181; misuse of 119, 120
Behaviour therapy 178, 179
Benzhexol 182
Bethlehem hospital 12
Brain damage 105; and subnormality 143
Brietal 186

Cannabis 120
Catatonic schizophrenia 82, 83
Catatonic stupor 82, 83
Causation, *see* mental illness
Chemotherapy 180–5
Childbirth and mental illness 54

Child, development of 19–23
Chloral hydrate 181
Chlordiazepoxide 182
Chlorpromazine 181, 182
Classification, *see* mental disorder, mental illness
Clomipramine 183
Cocaine, misuse of 121
Community care: of mentally ill 194–6; of mentally subnormal 146–8
Community psychiatric nurse 196
Compulsions 41, 62
Conditioning 178
Confabulation 99
Confused patients, management of 100–2
Confusion 46; acute 103–5, case illustration 109–10; chronic 105, 106
Connolly, J. 13
Consciousness, clouding of 104
Conversion 36
Cretinism 145
Crime and mental illness 156–8

Day hospital 196
Defence mechanisms, *see* mental mechanisms
Delirium, *see* confusion, acute
Delirium tremens 127
Delusions: hypochondriacal 43, 44, 78, 79; nihilistic 44 79, 81; of grandeur 43; of guilt and unworthiness 44, 79; of poverty 44, 78; paranoid 43, 81, 83, 84, 99
Dementia 98; arteriosclerotic 103; presenile 102, 103; senile 98–102, case illustration 106–9
Depixol 182
Depression 42; endogenous 77, 78, case illustration 88–90; reactive 63, 64, case illustration 72, 73
Desensitisation 178
Diazepam 182
Dichloralphenazone 181
Disablement resettlement officer 194
Disorientation 46; in senile dementia 99
Dissociation 36
Down's disease, *see* mongolism
Doxepin 183
Drug dependence 117–32

Echolalia 41
Echopraxia 41
Elation 41, 42
Electro-convulsive therapy 15, 185–9; preparation of patient for 186; unilateral 188, 189
Electroencephalogram 138
Emotion, inappropriate 42; lability of 42
Employment service agency 194
Endogenous depression 77, 78
Epilepsy 133–40; and mental illness 136; anticonvulsant treatment of 138, 139; idiopathic 133; Jacksonian, 135, 137; symptomatic 133; temporal lobe 135, 138
Epileptic fit: major 134, 136, 137; minor 135, 137
Epileptic patients: management of 139, 140; problems of 139
Extroverts 26

Fetishism 155, 156
Fits, *see* epileptic fit; withdrawal 122
Freud, S. 15, 34, 35, 177
Frigidity 154
Fugues 61

General paralysis of the insane 14
Government training centre 194
Grandeur, delusions of 43
Group homes 195
Gustatory hallucinations 45

Hallucinations: auditory 45, 81; gustatory 45; olfactory 45; tactile 45; visual 45, 80, 81, 83
Haloperidol 182
Hebephrenic schizophrenia 83
Heredity and mental illness 51
Homosexuality 154, 155; in adolescence 24
Hostels 147, 195
Human development 19, 30
Huntington's chorea 102
Hydrocephalus 146
Hypnosis 177, 178
Hypnotics 180, 181
Hypochondriacal delusions 43, 44, 78, 79
Hypochondriacal features, in anxiety 58
Hypomania 75–7, case illustration 86–8
Hysteria 60, 61, case illustration 70–2; personality in 61

Illusions 46, 104
Imipramine 183

Immaturity, emotional 26, 27
Impotence 154
Industrial therapy 192
Insomnia 39
Institutionalism 167–73
Insulin coma therapy 15
Intelligence 142
Introverts 26
Involutional melancholia 79

Jacksonian epilepsy 135, 137

Korsakov's psychosis 127

Lithium carbonate 76
Lorazepam 182
L.S.D., misuse of 121, 122
Malarial therapy 15
Mania 75–7
Manic-depressive psychosis 75
Masocism 156
Maturation 20–1
Mental disorder, classification of 47
Mental Health Acts 16
Mental illness: causes of 50–5; classification of 47, 48
Mental mechanisms 35–7
Mental subnormality, *see* subnormality
Mescaline, misuse of 121, 122
Mesmer, F. 177
Methadone 124
Microcephalus 145, 146
Middle age 28; and mental illness 54
Mind: censor in 35; conscious 34; preconscious 34; unconscious 34–7
Modecate 86, 182
Moditen 86, 182
Mongolism 144, 145
Monoamine oxidase inhibitors 183
Murder and mental illness 158

Negativism 41
Neologisms 44
Neuroses 48, 56–73; classification of 57
Neurotic personality 56
Nialamide 183
Nihilistic delusion 44, 79, 81
Nitrazepam 181

Obesity 152, 153
Obsessional fears 62, 63
Obsessions 44, 62
Obsessive-compulsive neurosis 62, 63; case illustration 68–70

Occupational therapy 191, 192
Old age 29–32; problems of 30–1
Old people, help for 31, 32
Olfactory hallucinations 45
Opiates, misuse of 121
Orphenadrine 182
Overactive patients, management of 76, 77
Overactivity 40, 76

Paedophilia 155
Panic attack 58
Paranoia 83, 84
Paranoid delusions 43, 81, 83, 84, 99
Paranoid schizophrenia 83
Paraphrenia 83
Parkinsonian symptoms, drug induced 181, 182
Pathological lying 111
Peptic ulcer 152
Perphenazine 181
Phenelzine 183
Phenobarbitone 138
Phenylketonuria 145
Phenytoin 138
Phobias 44, 45, 60
Phobic anxiety 60, case illustration 66–8
Pinel, P. 13
Pre-senile dementias 102, 103
Primidone 138
Procyclidine 182
Projection 37
Promazine 181
Psychiatric hospital, functions of 16–18
Psychoanalysis 177
Psychological development, *see* human development
Psychoneuroses, *see* neuroses
Psychopathic disorder, 47, 111–14, case illustration 114–16
Psychopathic patients, management of 113, 114
Psychoses 48; functional 75–96; organic 98–110
Psychosomatic disorders 150–3
Psychotherapy 175, 176
Puberty 23–4

Quinalbarbitone 180

Rationalisation 36, 37
Reaction formation 36
Reactive depression 63, 64
Recreational therapy 193, 194
Regression 37; in children 21

Rehabilitation 190–6
Repression 36
Retardation 40

Sadism 156
Schizophrenia 79–86; case illustrations 90–6; catatonic 82, 83; hebephrenic 83; paranoid 83; simple 81, 82
Scoline 186, 187
Seclusion of patients 162
Senile dementia 98–102
Sexual offences 157
Sexual problems 153–6
Sheltered workshop 147, 195
Shoplifting and mental illness 157
Simple schizophrenia 81, 82
Social worker 32, 196
Special care unit 147
Special hospital 16, 158
Status epilepticus 135, 137, 138
Stupor 41; catatonic 82
Sublimation 36
Subnormality 47, 142–9; causes of 142, 143; severe 47, 144; treatment of, 146–9
Suicidal gestures 164
Suicide 163–5; in endogenous depression 78; in reactive depression 63; precautions 164–5
Sulthiame 138

Tactile hallucinations 45
Temporal lobe epilepsy 135, 138
Therapeutic community 17
Thioridazine 181
Thought blocking 44
Token economy 179
Tranquillizers 181, 182
Transference 177
Transvestism 155
Treatment: physical 180–9; psychological 175–9
Triclofos 181
Trifluoperazine 181

Ulcerative colitis 152
Unconscious mind 34–7

Violent behaviour 157; management of 161, 162
Visual hallucinations 45, 80, 81, 83
Voyeurism 156

Withdrawal symptoms 122, 123